AF735609

CANCER ETIOLOGY, DIAGNOSIS AND TREATMENTS

NEW DEVELOPMENTS IN ONCOLOGY RESEARCH

Cancer Etiology, Diagnosis and Treatments

Additional books and e-books in this series can be found on Nova's website under the Series tab.

CANCER ETIOLOGY, DIAGNOSIS AND TREATMENTS

NEW DEVELOPMENTS IN ONCOLOGY RESEARCH

MARCOS T. BLAIR
EDITOR

nova
Medicine & Health
New York

Copyright © 2019 by Nova Science Publishers, Inc.

All rights reserved. No part of this book may be reproduced, stored in a retrieval system or transmitted in any form or by any means: electronic, electrostatic, magnetic, tape, mechanical photocopying, recording or otherwise without the written permission of the Publisher.

We have partnered with Copyright Clearance Center to make it easy for you to obtain permissions to reuse content from this publication. Simply navigate to this publication's page on Nova's website and locate the "Get Permission" button below the title description. This button is linked directly to the title's permission page on copyright.com. Alternatively, you can visit copyright.com and search by title, ISBN, or ISSN.

For further questions about using the service on copyright.com, please contact:
Copyright Clearance Center
Phone: +1-(978) 750-8400 Fax: +1-(978) 750-4470 E-mail: info@copyright.com.

NOTICE TO THE READER

The Publisher has taken reasonable care in the preparation of this book, but makes no expressed or implied warranty of any kind and assumes no responsibility for any errors or omissions. No liability is assumed for incidental or consequential damages in connection with or arising out of information contained in this book. The Publisher shall not be liable for any special, consequential, or exemplary damages resulting, in whole or in part, from the readers' use of, or reliance upon, this material. Any parts of this book based on government reports are so indicated and copyright is claimed for those parts to the extent applicable to compilations of such works.

Independent verification should be sought for any data, advice or recommendations contained in this book. In addition, no responsibility is assumed by the Publisher for any injury and/or damage to persons or property arising from any methods, products, instructions, ideas or otherwise contained in this publication.

This publication is designed to provide accurate and authoritative information with regard to the subject matter covered herein. It is sold with the clear understanding that the Publisher is not engaged in rendering legal or any other professional services. If legal or any other expert assistance is required, the services of a competent person should be sought. FROM A DECLARATION OF PARTICIPANTS JOINTLY ADOPTED BY A COMMITTEE OF THE AMERICAN BAR ASSOCIATION AND A COMMITTEE OF PUBLISHERS.

Additional color graphics may be available in the e-book version of this book.

Library of Congress Cataloging-in-Publication Data

ISBN: 978-1-53615-365-1

Published by Nova Science Publishers, Inc. † New York

CONTENTS

PREFACE

In the opening chapter, authors discuss the current literature that describes the application of Palliative Medicine services in advanced cancer, models of Palliative Care delivery by site and mode of practice, cost-effectiveness of early Palliative Medicine referral patterns and national and international Palliative Medicine practice and referral guidelines. The chapter will also discuss the outcomes of Palliative Medicine in Oncology focusing on the improvements in patient clinical and quality of life outcomes.

Next, a systematic chapter aims to better explain the mechanisms that underlie electrolyte disturbances in cancer patients, to stress on the serious prognostic implications involved and to provide practical and useful indications for the prompt diagnosis, management and therapy of electrolyte disorders.

The authors discuss over thirty Pt{η2-P(X)nP}Cl2 (n = 5,6,7,8) derivatives in which organodiphosphines create wide varieties of the metallocyclic rings: eight-membered (PC5P, PC2OC2P, PC2NC2P), nine-membered (PC6P, POC4OP), ten-membered (POC5OP, PC2OCOC2P, PC3OC3P), and eleven-membered (PC8P, PNC6NP, POC6OP). Another included study covers eighty five Pt(II) complexes with an inner coordination sphere of cis- PtP2Cl2. The P- donor ligands are organodiphosphines which create four- and five-membered metallocyclic rings with the PCP, PNP, PC-CP, PC=CP, PN2P and PCOP types. In the penultimate chapter, the authors examine over forty cis-Pt(η2-PXXXP)Cl2 derivatives in which organodiphosphines create six-membered metallocyclic rings, and the concluding chapter examines over thirty cis-Pt(η2-PXXXXP)Cl2 derivatives in which organodihosphines create seven-membered metallocyclic rings.

Chapter 1 - Palliative Medicine has a far-reaching role in the continuum of comprehensive cancer treatment and complete oncology patient care. The multidisciplinary teams of Palliative Medicine and Oncology serve a combined function of providing primary and secondary Palliative Care for treatment of difficult patient symptoms and maintaining patient quality of life by defining patient goals of care. Despite years of clear evidence and the recognition by oncologic societies of the fundamental need to integrate the specialties of Palliative Medicine and Oncology, the assimilation of these practices remains challenging. In this chapter, the authors discuss the current literature that describes the application of Palliative Medicine services in advanced cancer, models of Palliative Care delivery by site and mode of practice, cost-effectiveness of early Palliative Medicine referral patterns and national and international Palliative Medicine practice and referral guidelines. The chapter will also discuss the outcomes of Palliative Medicine in Oncology focusing on the improvements in patient clinical and quality of life outcomes. Additionally, Palliative Medicine provides patient distress relief, family and caregiver support, and reinforces the importance of advance care planning. Adaptation of Palliative Medicine in Oncology has proven to improve patient outcomes and decrease healthcare costs, supporting the national guidelines and recommendations for early involvement of Palliative Medicine at the time of or shortly after a cancer diagnosis. There are additional guidelines to assist in identifying patients at hospital admission for Palliative Care consultation. The chapter will explore barriers to these practice recommendations including an undersupplied Palliative Medicine workforce and deficient understanding of the roles of Palliative Medicine by patients and oncologists. The chapter concludes with expert commentary regarding forthcoming areas of Palliative Care in

Oncology that need further exploration and potential directions for future research and practice models.

Chapter 2 - Electrolyte disorders are common in cancer patients and can determine a worsening prognosis. However, these alterations are often misunderstood or not considered in clinical practice. The most common electrolyte alterations involve sodium, potassium, calcium and magnesium serum level. These electrolyte disorders might be related either to cancer physiopathology (e.g., paraneoplastic syndromes such as the syndrome of inappropriate secretion of ADH-SIADH, tumor lysis syndrome, etc.), or anti-cancer agents or other concomitant treatments. Moreover, they are often multifactorial or can result from comorbidities or unknown causes. Electrolyte disorders might cause life-threatening morbidity causing multiple organ systems dysfunction. Furthermore, emerging data showed that they might influence cancer patients' outcome, whether not promptly corrected. In particular, they seem to be correlated with poorer performance status, they might cause delays in therapy and negatively affect treatments' response and survival. Therefore, it is necessary to better understand the physiological principles underlying these disorders and at the same time to achieve an early identification, in order to attempt an adequate and effective therapy and an appropriate monitoring. This systematic review aims to better explain the mechanisms that underlie electrolyte disturbances in cancer patients, to stress on the serious prognostic implications involved and to provide practical and useful indications for the prompt diagnosis, management and therapy of electrolyte disorders.

Chapter 3 - This review includes over thirty $Pt\{\eta^2\text{-}P(X)_nP\}Cl_2$ ($n = 5, 6, 7, 8$) derivatives in which organodiphosphines create wide varieties of the metallocyclic rings: eight-membered (PC_5P, PC_2OC_2P, PC_2NC_2P), nine-membered (PC_6P, POC_4OP), ten-membered (POC_5OP, PC_2OCOC_2P, PC_3OC_3P), and eleven-membered (PC_8P, PNC_6NP, POC_6OP). In those derivatives the most common is a predominantly cis-arrangement (31 examples) and only 3 examples with trans-configuration. The total mean values of Pt-L bond distances in the complexes (cis- vs trans-configuration) are: 2.232 Å (L = P), 2.353 Å (L = Cl) vs 2.312 and 2.307 Å, respectively. These data are compared and discussed with those found in cis-PtP_2Cl_2

derivatives of Pt{η^2-P(X)$_n$P}Cl_2 (n = 1,2,3,4) types. Two complexes exist in two isomeric forms cis- and trans-..

Chapter 4 - This review covers eighty five Pt(II) complexes with an inner coordination sphere of cis-PtP_2Cl_2. The P-donor ligands are organodiphosphines which create four- and five-membered metallocyclic rings with the PCP, PNP, PC-CP, PC=CP, PN_2P and PCOP types. The effects of both steric and electronic factors can be seen from the values of the P-Pt-P bite angles, with the mean values: 74.4° (PCP), 71.8° (PNP), 87.3° (PC-CP), 86.5° (PC=CP), 84.3° (PN_2P) and 84.0° (PCOP). The mean value of Pt-P bond distance of 2.217 Å (trans to Cl) is much shorter (more covalent) than the mean value of Pt-Cl bond distance of 2.364 Å (trans to P), as a reason of stronger trans- influence of P over Cl. There are complexes which are examples of distortion and ligand isomerism.

Chapter 5 - This review includes over forty cis-Pt(η^2-PXXXP)Cl_2 derivatives in which organodiphosphines create six-membered metallocyclic rings. There are wide varieties of the respective rings of the types: PC_3P (most common), PCNCP, PCSCP, PCSiCP, PNCNP, PCCOP, PCCNP, POPNP, POSiOP and P(XXX)$_2$P. The total mean values of Pt-P and Pt-Cl bond distances are 2.222 Å and 2.358 Å. The total mean values of the bite P-Pt-P bond angles is 94.0°. These data are compared and discussed with those found in cis-PtP_2Cl_2 derivatives of Pt(η^2-PXP)(Cl)$_2$ and Pt(η^2-PX_2P)(Cl)$_2$ types. There are complexes which are examples of distortion isomerism.

Chapter 6 - This review includes over thirty cis-Pt(η^2-PXXXXP)Cl_2 derivatives in which organodihosphines create seven- membered metallocyclic rings. There are five varieties of the respective rings of the types: PC_4P (most common), POC_2OP, PNC_2NP, PSC_2SP and PNC_2OP. The mean values of Pt-P and Pt-Cl bond distances are 2.239 Å and 2.346 Å, respectively. The mean values of cis-L-Pt-L bond angles open in the sequence: 87.3° (Cl-Pt-Cl) < 87.7° (P-Pt-Cl) < 96.8° (P-Pt-P). The mean value of trans-P-Pt-Cl bond angle is 173.5°. These data are compared and discussed with those found in cis-PtP_2Cl_2 derivatives of Pt(η^2-PXP)(Cl)$_2$, Pt(η^2-PXXP)(Cl)$_2$ and Pt(η^2-PXXXXP)(Cl)$_2$ types. There are complexes which are examples of distortion isomerism.

In: New Developments in Oncology Research ISBN: 978-1-53615-365-1
Editor: Marcos T. Blair © 2019 Nova Science Publishers, Inc.

Chapter 1

PALLIATIVE CARE IN ONCOLOGY

Laura Finn, MD[1] and Sonia Malhotra, MD[2]
[1]Division of Hematology and Bone Marrow Transplant,
Department of Internal Medicine, Ochsner Medical Center,
New Orleans, Louisiana, US
[2]Department of Palliative Medicine and Supportive Care,
Section of General Internal Medicine and Geriatrics,
University Medical Center/Tulane University School of Medicine,
New Orleans, Louisiana, US

ABSTRACT

Palliative Medicine has a far-reaching role in the continuum of comprehensive cancer treatment and complete oncology patient care. The multidisciplinary teams of Palliative Medicine and Oncology serve a combined function of providing primary and secondary Palliative Care for treatment of difficult patient symptoms and maintaining patient quality of life by defining patient goals of care. Despite years of clear evidence and the recognition by oncologic societies of the fundamental need to integrate the specialties of Palliative Medicine and Oncology, the assimilation of these practices remains challenging. In this chapter, we discuss the current literature that describes the application of Palliative Medicine services in advanced cancer, models of Palliative Care delivery by site and mode of practice, cost-effectiveness of early Palliative Medicine referral patterns and national and international Palliative Medicine practice and referral guidelines. The chapter will also discuss the outcomes of Palliative Medicine in Oncology focusing on the improvements in patient clinical and quality of life outcomes. Additionally, Palliative Medicine provides patient distress relief, family and caregiver support, and reinforces the importance of advance care planning. Adaptation of Palliative Medicine in Oncology has proven to improve patient outcomes and decrease healthcare costs, supporting the national guidelines and recommendations for early involvement of Palliative Medicine at the time of or shortly after a cancer diagnosis. There are additional guidelines to assist in identifying patients at hospital admission for Palliative Care consultation. The chapter will explore barriers to these practice recommendations including an undersupplied Palliative Medicine workforce and deficient understanding of the roles of Palliative Medicine by patients and oncologists. The chapter concludes with expert commentary regarding forthcoming areas of Palliative Care in Oncology that need further exploration and potential directions for future research and practice models.

Keywords: cancer pain, cost-benefit analysis, medical oncology, surgical oncology, palliative medicine

1. Introduction

1.1. Defining Palliative Medicine

Palliative Care and its medical subspecialty known as Palliative Medicine is the specialized care of people living with serious illness including cancer. The medical specialty focuses on alleviating the burden of difficult symptoms and improving patient quality of life [1]. It is appropriate for any age and any stage of serious illness and is ideally provided concurrently with curative and life prolonging treatments. Palliative Medicine specialists work alongside a patient's team of providers to deliver symptom treatment and communication expertise, emotional support, assistance with medical decision making, along with assistance with end of life care and bereavement support when appropriate. Core palliative medicine teams may consist of physicians, advanced practice providers, nurses, social workers and chaplains. Other providers such as psychologists, pharmacists, child life specialists, music and art therapists are often utilized as part of the multidisciplinary Palliative Medicine team for specific aspects of patient care.

Early introduction to palliative medicine can effectively improve quality of life for patients with cancer. A landmark study in the field of palliative medicine evaluated patients with metastatic non-small-cell lung cancer and randomized patients into two groups of either standard oncology care versus same oncology care with the addition of outpatient Palliative Medicine consultations and follow-up visits. The patients randomized to Palliative Medicine had improved quality of life scores, improved anxiety screening scores, and improved depression screening scores. Additionally, patients in the Palliative Medicine group had decreased percentages of patient deaths in the hospital, less aggressive end-of-life care, and higher rates of resuscitation status preference documentation or advanced care planning. Interestingly, a secondary outcome of improved median overall survival was noted in the patients receiving the Palliative Care intervention (11.6 vs 8.9 months) [2].

Patient and family support is an essential component of the practice of Palliative Medicine. From a medical standpoint, Palliative Medicine teams can provide patients with effective pain and symptom management even in the most complex of symptom cases. From a communication standpoint, Palliative Care supports patients with medical decision making as well as team cohesion and treatment recommendations when presented to patients and families. Patients and families often have higher rates of satisfaction with their medical care and the quality of communication when Palliative Medicine teams are involved [3]. Early Palliative Medicine involvement can help families feel less angry and less in denial about the anticipated death of their loved one [4]. Palliative medicine teams also help patients and families as they transition to end-of-life and often assist with bereavement support.

1.2. Primary vs Secondary and Tertiary Palliative Care

The application of Palliative Care services may be distributed among primary Palliative Care providers and secondary providers that work together and form a multidisciplinary team. Oncologists, psychologists/ psychiatrists, surgeons, radiation oncologists, and primary care physicians are only a few of the types of clinicians who provide primary Palliative Care for initial symptom control including management of pain and non-pain symptoms related to a diagnosis of cancer or its treatments such as surgery, radiation therapy, stem cell transplants and/or cancer survivorship. The approach to primary symptom therapy involves the entire oncology multidisciplinary care team. Often the first application of primary Palliative Care is either treatment of the symptoms of cancer or of adverse side effects from treatment with the most common symptom being pain. The National Cancer Care Network published its latest guidelines in 2018 for managing adult cancer pain which includes recommendations for performing a comprehensive pain assessment and utilizing a pain intensity rating scale, use of non-opioid therapies, initiating short and long acting opioid medications, and integrative interventions [5]. More challenging side effects may be encountered with the use of immunotherapies which are becoming standard of care for many malignancies. Use of immune therapy requires knowledge of the potential side effects and early recognition for rapid initiation of therapy [6]. Additional guidelines are also available for primary Palliative Care in Oncology for the treatment of emesis including differentiating symptom treatment amongst the emetic potential of treatment regimens, anticipatory emesis and refractory nausea and vomiting [7]. Recommendations are available for assessment and treatment of cancer related fatigue including screening for compounding factors such as depression or substance abuse, evaluation of comorbid conditions and treatment of anemia, sleep disturbances and nutritional deficiencies that may result from the underlying cancer or therapies used to treat it [8]. Identifying psychosocial and spiritual distress requires asking difficult questions at time of diagnosis and throughout the course of cancer treatment. Distress management includes use of the multidisciplinary team which includes mental health professionals for emotional distress, social workers for social and home distress and chaplaincy care for spiritual distress which is discussed further in this chapter [9].

Secondary Palliative Care is specialty level management provided by teams of Palliative Medicine providers who build upon the care already provided during primary Palliative Care services [10, 11]. Adding specialty Palliative Care further enhances the multidisciplinary team and addresses the patient's needs beyond basic symptom management and includes the management of more difficult to manage symptoms, psychosocial needs, caregiver stewardship and setting goals of care with additional advanced care planning. A parallel example to this can be seen when patients with coronary artery disease are admitted and evaluated as to whether or not they should be seen by a cardiologist and admitted to a cardiac care unit. Similarly, not all patients with a cancer diagnosis need a Palliative Care consult, however many require this level of secondary specialty management. Qualitative studies report that patients can easily discern the distinct roles held by their Oncologist who is providing cancer therapy and their Palliative Medicine clinician who is providing symptom control and emotional support [12]. Studies also show that oncology patients may prefer to discuss end of life issues, goals of care and advance care planning with a physician other than their Oncologist [13]. It has been demonstrated that patients accept Palliative Medicine without "loss of hope" which has been a documented concern of many Oncologists. The data to support this should serve to inform clinicians that there is no reason to avoid Palliative Medicine consultations until failure of therapy, symptom crises, or end of life [14, 15]. The concept of tertiary Palliative Medicine is more often provided at academic medical centers that have large groups of Palliative Medicine specialists who perform research to advance the field and care for more highly complex patients [16]. Secondary and tertiary Palliative Care can facilitate treatment of challenging symptoms of cancer including refractory or atypical pain, cancer fatigue and anorexia.

1.3. Symptom Management

1.3.1. Special Issues in Hematologic Malignancies

Patients with hematologic disorders and malignancies represent a unique patient population often dependent on transfusion of blood products for prolongation of life and improved quality of physical and mental life. Studies show that in the last 30 days of life, patients with hematologic malignancies have an increased number of emergency room visits, hospital admissions, intensive care unit admissions and hospital deaths compared to patients with solid organ malignancies. These patients have fewer Palliative Care unit admissions, inpatient Palliative Care service consults and outpatient Palliative Care service consults [17]. Patients with hematologic malignancies are often dependent on blood transfusions to control the symptoms of their diseases and are less likely to use Palliative Medicine services and hospice, often due to a false belief by many referring physicians that blood transfusions are not allowed within the Medicare hospice benefit [18]. When patients with the end stages of leukemia enroll in hospice care services, the negative outcomes of poor end-of-life care improve significantly and overall costs may be reduced for Medicare beneficiaries by up to 15,000 dollars per patient in the last month of life. The financial barrier to Palliative Medicine consultation and referral to hospice care for these patients is the low per diem reimbursement provided to hospices by Medicare, restricting palliative-intent blood transfusions because of cost, though the cost of this intervention is relatively low. Studies have shown that Hematologists would refer more patients to Palliative Medicine and hospice if red blood cell and platelet transfusions could be provided for palliative symptom control [19].

1.4. Distress Relief

1.4.1. Physical Distress

A 2017 systematic review showed that early Palliative Care intervention in patients with advanced cancer has beneficial effects on quality of life and symptom intensity [20]. Palliative care intervention for physical symptoms due to cancer, cancer therapies and comorbid conditions is not limited to the treatment of pain. Other physical symptoms include fatigue, nausea and vomiting, anorexia, anxiety and depression and neuropathies. The treatment of emesis has published guidelines including grading systems that predict the potential of chemotherapy to cause nausea and the treatment of anticipatory or delayed nausea and vomiting. An area of improvement needed in primary Palliative Care is the standardization of the treatment of emesis. Oncologists need to be well versed in the treatment of chemotherapy related nausea however studies of adherence to antiemetic guidelines demonstrate highly variable practice patterns [21, 22].

Pain management is another area that needs improvement among primary Palliative Care providers. One such study demonstrating this compared the practice of Oncologists to Palliative Medicine clinicians at pain management. This study found that Oncologists had many difficulties when managing challenging pain scenarios and yet rated their own abilities to do this much higher than outcomes reported [23]. Gaps in pain management education in Oncology are clearly identified, suggesting Palliative Medicine consultations may be needed more frequently for this particular symptom.

Many bone marrow transplant programs have harnessed the relief of physical distress by incorporating Palliative Care specialists, creating unique interdisciplinary teams for the treatment of hematologic cancers. Symptoms of hematologic cancers include pain, dyspnea, fatigue, mucositis, diarrhea, anorexia and delirium. Furthermore, the risk of death from the underlying hematologic malignancy is exacerbated by the mortality related to transplant. Palliative Care physicians incorporated into transplant programs report pain management being the most common symptom they were asked to address. A study at Western Pennsylvania Hospital demonstrated that 66% of bone marrow transplant patients receiving consultation for pain control reported relief within 48 hours of consultation. Additionally, goals of care documentation occurred in 67% of patients and hospice referrals increased from 5% to 41% in patients at the end-of-life during the study period. This same study showed that 100% of bone marrow transplant physicians were extremely satisfied with their experience with Palliative Medicine [24]. A separate study at the University of California San Francisco showed improvement in dyspnea scores with Palliative Care consultation in patients with advanced cancer, emphysema or congestive heart failure when compared to a control group with usual care. Improvements were also seen in anxiety, sleep quality and spiritual well-being in the Palliative Care intervention group [25]. Patients in the New Hampshire Project ENABLE (Educate, Nurture, Advise, Before Life Ends) study randomized patients with advanced gastrointestinal, lung, genitourinary tract and breast cancer to psychoeducational interventions with Palliative Care advanced practice providers. When compared to those with usual care, the Palliative Care intervention group reported improvements in patient quality of life, symptom intensity and mood [26].

1.4.2. Emotional Distress

Virtually all patients with cancer and those facing a terminal diagnosis experience sadness. A component of sadness is grief which is defined as the emotion or reaction in response to loss. The diagnosis of advanced cancer may surface this feeling of loss which includes loss of identity, independence, occupation and the social support system including family. The grief patients feel may be multi-factorial and include social, emotional, spiritual and physical changes. The physical and psychological burdens felt by patients with advanced cancer can be substantial with significant reports of pain and loss of dignity [27]. Preparatory grief is a distinct process that terminally ill patients experience to prepare for separation from the world as described by Dr. Kubler-Ross in her landmark publication “On Death and Dying.” This is distinctly different from anticipatory grief which is the feeling family and friends have before the loss of a loved one [28]. The sadness patients experience may manifest in degrees beyond simple grief. Included in this is complicated grief which is defined as a prolonged grief disorder that lasts more than 6 months. Mental health illnesses such as depression and anxiety may also present [29]. Manifestations of sadness beyond simple grief are important to identify as they predict poorer patient quality of life and development of mental illness [30]. The differentiation between preparatory grief and depression can be difficult due the presentation of similar symptoms but is essential due to the impact of therapeutic implications.

Grief is a well described system of reactions to deal with loss that does not respond well to biochemical intervention. In contrast, depression may occur alongside grief and is distinguished by its symptomatology which can include feelings of sadness, poor sleep, changes in appetite, low interest, decreased concentration, feelings of worthlessness and possible suicidal ideations that impact functioning. The best evidence for depression management involves the combination of behavioral counseling and medical therapies such as antidepressants [31]. Some symptoms of preparatory grief and depression may overlap and these include appetite and weight changes, fatigue and sleep disturbances [27]. Symptoms of depression further include anhedonia, hopelessness, disturbed self-esteem, persistent thoughts of suicide and possibly a desire for an early death. A 2017 randomized control trial demonstrated that early Palliative Care interventions with in-person consultation and nurse facilitated phone sessions impact patient's depressive symptoms and can decrease patient mortality risk scores [32]. The monitoring for grief disorders and depression is equally as important for caregivers and bereaved family members. Symptoms of depression among bereaved family members, especially spouses, rate as high as 73% in the first month after the loss and decrease over 2 years to about 15% [33, 34]. Predictors of complicated grief and symptoms of depression among the bereaved include severe preparatory grief, prior depression and lower levels of education [33]. Palliative Care and mental health professionals are vital to providing therapy for complicated emotional distress in patients, caregivers and family members.

1.4.3. Spiritual Distress

Spirituality may be defined as "the aspect of humanity that refers to the way individuals seek and express meaning and purpose and the way they experience their connectedness to the moment, to self, to others, to nature and to the significant or sacred" [35]. Spirituality may be a critical component to the care of patients with advanced cancer and those at the end-of-life. Evidence shows that spiritual support is associated with better quality of care, less aggressive care at the end-of-life and increased hospice use [36]. The value of being aware of a patient's spiritual needs can result in more effective communication regarding goals of care. This awareness allows the health care team to honor personal values and end-of-life wishes. It can also help establish trust with clinicians providing oncologic and palliative care treatments [37]. One study examined advanced cancer patients receiving palliative radiation therapy and their views regarding spirituality and the perception of its importance to the attention of health care clinicians. Over 80% of participants relied on their religion and spirituality to cope with their cancer and felt it improved their quality of life. These same participants thought clinicians' attention to their spirituality was an important part of their cancer care [38]. A Spanish study of cancer patients receiving palliative treatment reported high quality of life among those with high use of spiritual coping [39]. Increased awareness of spirituality is important and can lend credence to consulting Palliative Care to help in addressing this.

Spiritual pain can be defined as the "pain caused by extinction of the being and the meaning of self "[40]. Several studies at MD Anderson have found that nearly half of patients report spiritual pain during their care and this adversely affects physical and emotional well-being. Spiritual pain was associated with increased depression, anxiety, anorexia and fatigue [41, 42]. Reports of negative spiritual coping and thoughts of punishment or abandonment by God were more highly associated with depression and adverse physical and emotional well-being [43]. Palliative Care clinicians are trained to assess for spiritual distress through spiritual screenings. Additionally, Palliative Medicine being a multidisciplinary specialty often includes chaplains, many of whom are board certified, to provide spiritual care specialty consultations. Use of spiritual care services becomes increasingly important during the disease trajectory of patients with a poor prognosis associated with their advanced cancer. This ensures that patients at the end-of-life won't have spiritual emergencies and instead have a meaningful, patient-centered dying experience.

1.5. Family and Caregiver Support

Caregivers are an under acknowledged, yet essential resource the in the care of oncology patients throughout the continuum of their care. There is a growing need to address the long-term well-being of caregivers. The diagnosis of advanced or terminal cancer and confrontation with mortality becomes a crisis on many levels for patients and their support systems. Caregivers assist with activities of daily living (ADL's), transportation, medications, finances, emotional support and serve as advocate for the health care of the patient. The list of ADL's includes and is not limited to eating, bathing, dressing, toileting, walking, and continence.[44] Approximately 50% of caregivers who assist with all six activities report difficulty with these tasks [45]. Personal care activities requiring a greater deal of physical stress such as feeding, bathing and toileting are reported to be most difficult [46]. Caregivers can spend 40 hours or more per week providing these services which can lead to increased distress manifesting as decreased physical wellbeing [47-50]. Patients and caregivers experience the emotions of a cancer diagnosis and require psychological care from diagnosis through survival or salvage care. Symptoms of stress experienced during the cancer diagnosis and treatment include exhaustion, social isolation and financial toxicity that may last for years [51]. The degree of emotional distress experienced by caregivers of bone marrow transplant patients has been reported to equal that of psychiatric inpatients [52, 53]. Palliative Care services are vital to providing caregiver support. In the ENABLE III study, caregivers of oncology patients were randomized to early versus delayed Palliative Medicine counseling. Caregivers receiving early counseling had decreased rates of depression and improved quality of life [54]. Early inclusion of Palliative Medicine can facilitate better communication among the patient-caregiver dyad and among patients, caregivers and the healthcare team, decreasing caregiver burden. When timing is appropriate and patients have elected to forego treatment options or exhausted them, hospice can add an additional layer of support and bereavement care for the families of patients.

1.6. Advance Care Planning

The World Health Organization defines advance care planning as the process of "planning in advance for decisions that may have to be made prior to incapability or end of life" [55]. Advance directives are documents that communicate these wishes including health care power of attorney, living will and physician orders for life sustaining therapy. Advance directives became more prominent in healthcare during the 1970's when the case of Karen Ann Quinlan, a 21-year-old woman who was resuscitated after drug and alcohol induced cardiopulmonary arrest, was brought to public attention when her parents appealed and succeeded at removing ventilation through the New Jersey Supreme court. This brought the concept of the living will to light [56]. A living will is a written statement or advance directive of a person's wishes regarding their medical treatment when communication cannot occur and what is known as informed consent cannot occur. In 1983, 25-year-old Nancy Cruzan ended up in a persistent vegetative state after a motor vehicle accident. Five years into her condition her parents appealed to the United States Supreme Court to discontinue her nutrition feeding tube. The Supreme Court agreed that patient's medical power of attorneys and/or next of kin could refuse interventions if wishes were expressed by a written advanced directive [56]. The Patient Self Determination Act followed, requiring medical institutions to inform patients of their right to have advance directives [57]. These cases of young adults with sudden and devastating health changes highlight that advance directives are for everyone no matter age, health status or racial or cultural background and simply are not limited to cancer patients or those with terminal illness. Advance care planning, though, does play a more important role as health changes and can be more urgent in the setting of a diagnosis of cancer or other serious illness.

A critical component of advance care planning is the completion of advance directives. These directives are legal documents detailing various aspects of healthcare decision making including who a patient would choose to make medical decisions if they were unable to do so from the loss of capacity due to illness or injury. This is known as the healthcare power of attorney. A living will is a legal document that reflects choices for treatment in the event of a serious illness or injury. Often patients will list their resuscitation preferences in the living will as well as whether they would desire advanced interventions such as dialysis or artificial nutrition. In some states if a patient chooses to focus on comfort and foregoes cardiopulmonary resuscitation, a mobile document known at the Physician's Orders for Life Sustaining Treatment (POLST) can be filled out to reflect do not resuscitate/intubate (DNR/DNI) preferences. The discussions that lead to advance directives and their completion are vital to the entire healthcare team. These documents provide a legal framework to help establish patient's preferences, their wishes and goals of care in the event of a serious incident or should the patient be nearing the end-of-life. Research has demonstrated that patients who have advance directives have fewer intensive care admissions and hospital deaths, receive fewer life-prolonging measures and have increased use of hospice care resulting in improved quality of life [58, 59].

However, many patients with advanced cancer and their physicians do not discuss advance directives. This can lead to unwanted or futile care at the end of life and increase family distress if they are left to make difficult health care decisions as patients lose capacity to voice their own wishes. Research shows that less than 25% of patients admitted to the hospital with cancer have an advanced directive. Discussions regarding advance care planning may take place at any time. The ambulatory setting generally provides a better setting for patients to have these conversations to plan for the future while they are well enough to do so. Patients report lack of knowledge and procrastination as the two greatest barriers to completing advance directives. This indicates the importance of starting these conversations early and having them repeatedly throughout the disease and treatment trajectory. It is also important for clinicians to reiterate that patients discuss their wishes with family and caregivers. Up to one third of patients report that they have advance directives but have not discussed their end-of-life care preferences with anyone.[60] Additional research shows that advance care planning increases patient knowledge about options for goals of care and planning for end-of-life without decreasing hope or increasing anxiety, which should help lessen clinician distress to bring up these topics [61].

2. Models of Palliative Care Delivery

There is now a significant body of research, including several randomized control trials supporting concordant Palliative Care and Oncologic care compared to usual Oncologic care alone [62]. The question is now not whether Palliative Care is needed in Oncology but rather, what are the best models of delivery by care settings. National clinical practice guidelines published by the American Society of Clinical Oncology now state that concurrent Palliative Care with usual Oncology care is the standard of care and Palliative Medicine should become part of a patient's care team within 8 weeks of diagnosis of advanced cancer [63]. Palliative medicine can be provided in almost any care setting including inpatient hospital consultations, dedicated hospital based Palliative Medicine units, outpatient clinics, assisted living and long-term care facilities or even home-based care. The most familiar model of Palliative Medicine delivery is reported as inpatient consultative services which may include a single clinician, consultant Palliative Medicine interdisciplinary team, or a Palliative Medicine hospital unit [64]. Inpatient Palliative Medicine should be available for specialty consultation throughout the entire hospital setting from the emergency room to the intensive care unit. Outpatient Oncology access to Palliative Medicine is a priority as the majority of oncologic care is ambulatory. Due to challenges in implementation and the current Palliative Medicine workforce shortage, less than half of the nation's Palliative Medicine programs have outpatient services [65, 66]. Early interactions by Palliative Care can have preventative effects by avoiding escalation of symptoms during treatment or symptom crises at the end of life [67]. Early access to outpatient Palliative Medicine facilitates longitudinal care through the patient's cancer course, changing prognosis, and improves their transition of care through the spectrum of healthcare settings [68]. A single visit with a Palliative Medicine clinician will not fully address the needs of any patient. Inserting Palliative Medicine clinics within the ambulatory Oncology practice provides the advantages of increasing access to higher volumes of patients in need, facilitates early referrals and improves communication between the oncologist, other care team members and the Palliative Medicine team [69]. Integration of a pair of Palliative Care clinicians that included a physician and advanced practice practitioner into a private oncology practice decreased symptom burden by 21%, resulted in high satisfaction scores from the oncologist and increased Palliative Care clinic consultations by 87% over 2 years [69]. Project ENABLE showed that Palliative Medicine can be successfully implemented in a variety of oncology practice models including cancer centers, private oncology practices and rural clinics using a variety of patient encounters including individual consults and group meetings. It also showed that Palliative Medicine can be implemented at the time of advanced cancer diagnosis and that remote intervention by telemedicine is a feasible method of intervention [15]. The follow-up randomized control trial ENABLE II further tested the telemedicine model of intervention with successful improvement in patient quality of life. Patients had a lower risk of death in the year after trial enrollment (HR 0.67, 95% CI 0.496-0.906, $P = 0.009$) and had increased median survival when compared to controls with results of 14 vs 8.5 months ($p = 0.14$) [14]. When similar intervention was provided for caregivers of patients with advanced cancer in ENABLE III, caregivers in the intervention group had significantly lower depression scores and stress burden further supporting early Palliative Medicine consultations in Oncology [54].

2.1. Inpatient Palliative Care

The two primary models of inpatient Palliative Care seen are a) consultative services and b) inpatient units. In 2011, the percentage of hospitals with an inpatient Palliative Care service was 65% with hospitals with more than 300 beds representing more than 85% of programs with tertiary Palliative Care [70]. Factors associated with an increased likelihood of having hospital based Palliative Care services included not-for-profit institutions, institutions that owned a hospice program, status as an American College of Surgery approved cancer hospital and having a higher percentage of patients with a college education [70]. Palliative Medicine consultative teams provide expertise on symptom control, weigh in on specific questions for the referral including thoughts on goals of care and at some centers assume patient care. Generally inpatient Palliative Care units are found in larger hospitals or health care systems with the ability to admit patients for symptom management, support of severely distressed families or to manage the imminently dying patient. States ranking high with hospital-based Palliative Care demonstrated lower numbers of hospital deaths, decreased terminal hospital admissions and lower intensive care unit admissions during a patient's last 6 months of life which overall demonstrated improved quality and cost of care. A study of a high-volume, 11 bed, inpatient Palliative Care unit at Virginia Commonwealth University found that daily patient charges and cost of care was reduced by up to 74% as when compared to patients who died outside of the unit [71]. The inpatient Palliative Care unit at Mount Sinai hospital admitted over 1,000 patients within its first 2 years of opening and also demonstrated cost savings per patient when compared to the general hospital wards [72].

2.2. Outpatient Palliative Care

The primary practice of Oncology is either outpatient based with treatments provided in cancer and infusion centers or at home with oral targeted cancer agents. Consistent with this, most primary Palliative Care provided by oncologists is in the outpatient setting and consists of pain and symptom management. This has led to the demand for outpatient Palliative Care clinics, even those embedded in cancer centers. A study describing the incorporation of outpatient Palliative Care into a large private oncology system in Virginia found increased satisfaction with these services over the first 2 years of its inception and referrals increasing steadily by 87% in this time frame. These consultations saved Oncologists' time by addressing difficult goals of care conversations, difficult patient symptom burden and overall were associated with a decrease in reported symptoms by 21% [73]. Early outpatient Palliative Care referrals are also associated with fewer emergency room visits, less hospitalizations in the last 30 days of life and fewer hospital deaths. Outpatient Palliative Care is also associated with less aggressive end of life care [74]. Patients who utilize Palliative Care clinics are noted to have earlier referral and longer lengths of stay in hospice prior to death, providing patients and families with greater benefits to these services [75]. Outpatient Oncology practices may create practice pathways or automated formulas for patient referral. Other integrative models exist where Oncology and Palliative Care staff "huddle" to identify patients in need of Palliative Care services and plan shared Oncology-Palliative Care visits. A study of this model described a 10-fold increase in outpatient Palliative Care consults over 3 years with 97% of the Oncology practice patients having a Palliative Care consultation prior to death. A systematic review of criteria for outpatient Palliative Care consult identified 6 recurrent reasons for referral including cancer trajectory including overall prognosis, changing performance status, psychosocial distress and end-of-life care planning. Establishing a method to understand reasons to utilize outpatient Palliative Care clinics will help oncologists refer patients for earliest possible intervention, allow administrators to set benchmarks to assess program quality, allow for research of patient concerns and allow for development of clinical pathways [76].

3. Referral Patterns

It is important to dispel the myth commonly held by Oncologists that Palliative Medicine is only associated with end-of-life care [77]. Research supports a simple yet apparently effective measure in divesting the stigma of Palliative Care as end-of-life care by simply adding "supportive care" to the name of the Palliative Medicine team [78]. Palliative medicine teams titled "Palliative Medicine & Supportive Care" help surpass some of the barriers Oncologists demonstrate when referring patients despite numerous national guidelines [79-83]. The National Comprehensive Cancer Network has published criteria for patient referral to Palliative Medicine and includes patients with poor pain control, multiple allergies to pain medications, refractory non-pain symptoms, severe comorbidities and inability to complete advance care planning [84]. As previously discussed, clinical symptom and distress screening that triggers Palliative Medicine consults has strong potential to improve early referrals [85-87]. Cancer institutions and private practices need to set individual referral pathways to generate consults to the Palliative Care clinician and/or team to enhance the quality of primary Palliative Care services available and already being provided by Oncologists.

Palliative care referrals are not requested as often or as early as needed and the average referral of patients occurs late, generally 30-60 days before death. Families interviewed after the death of referred patients stated they desired earlier consultation [88-90]. Universal referral for all cancer patients is neither efficient nor feasible with the current Palliative Care workforce shortage. The majority of Palliative Care referrals currently are based on the judgement of the Oncologist or Cancer Team rather than patient need or standardized referral criteria [91]. When considering criteria, some possibilities such as the presence of metastatic or advanced cancer, poor functional status, one or more serious complications of cancer associated with prognosis of less than 1 year, presence of serious comorbid conditions or presence of persistent symptom distress may assist in standardizing referral criteria [92]. Patients with physical distress, especially pain are clear candidates for Palliative Care services [92, 93]. End-of-life care planning represents another common reason for referral and both inpatient and outpatient Palliative Care settings can facilitate these consultations. The need for end-of-life care planning should also be considered a standard trigger for referral [94]. Often patients who are admitted to the hospital for a cancer-related complication demonstrate need for a Palliative Medicine consult. A recent review of hospitalized patients shows that less than a third of those that meet standard criteria for specialty Palliative Care receive a request for Palliative Medicine consultation by their primary team [95, 96]. Younger Oncologists tend to have higher and earlier Palliative Care utilization and they refer patients at all stages, all ages (especially younger cancer patients) and utilize outpatient palliative services more often [96]. Outpatient Palliative Care clinics are becoming increasingly available. In 2009, 59% of the National Cancer Institute (NCI) designated cancer centers and 22% of non-NCI designated cancer centers reported these services [88]. Screening for referral to outpatient or inpatient Palliative Care is not a single time-point event and should be considered on a continual basis at every stage of disease.

4. Cost Effectiveness/Health System Considerations

Health care costs and utilization for patients with cancer, especially those with advanced cancer or at the end-of-life are significant since treatment trajectory often involves unexpected emergency room visits, hospital admissions, readmissions, futile and invasive procedures and intensive care utilization. A study recently identified a 75% increase in mortality in cancer patients within the year after an unexpected hospital admission [97]. Studies also show that readmission rates decrease significantly after Palliative Medicine consultation [98]. Patients with multiple co-morbidities account for a high proportion of health care utilization and spending. It has been estimated that direct hospital costs decrease by 22-32% when early Palliative Medicine consults are provided, namely within 2 days of admission for patients with co-morbidity scores of 2 or greater [99, 100]. Palliative Medicine consults provided within 6 days of hospital admission still provided a direct cost savings of approximately 14% [100-102]. Patients with early Palliative Medicine consultation are more likely to receive care outside of the intensive care unit, are less likely to be hospitalized repeatedly and enroll in hospice earlier [103]. Referral to outpatient Palliative Medicine clinics within 3 months of end-of-life also decreases hospital admission, decreases costs, increases hospice utilization and improves patient quality of life [104, 105]. The Centers for Medicare and Medicaid Services now provide separate payment for advance care planning discussions, an action that should promote earlier and increased Palliative Medicine consultations [106]. Appropriate use of Palliative Medicine services can yield institutional annual savings of nearly 2 million dollars by decreasing inpatient lengths of stay, reducing the hospital risk adjusted mortality index and lowering daily hospital costs [107, 108].

5. National Practice Guidelines and Society Recommendations

Evidence for synchronized efforts among Oncology and Palliative Medicine clinicians is very compelling and has led to guiding statements from prominent societies from both disciplines. In February of 2017, the American Society of Clinical Oncology (ASCO) updated their clinical practice guideline for the integration of Palliative Medicine into Oncology. ASCO recommends that all patients with advanced cancer receive Palliative Medicine services within 8 weeks of their diagnosis and concurrently with active inpatient or outpatient cancer treatment. Patient referrals to multidisciplinary Palliative Medicine teams are optimal. Advanced cancer is defined by ASCO as being those patients with metastatic disease, late-stage diagnosis and/or a prognosis of 24 months or less [109]. The Society of Gynecologic Oncology (SGO) recommends that primary Palliative Care for women with advanced or relapsed gynecologic cancer should not be delayed and timely referral be provided for secondary specialty Palliative Medicine [110]. The Society of Surgical Oncology has supported Palliative Medicine since 1998 stating "supportive care services and effective symptom management are essential to promoting the quality of life for people diagnosed with cancer. Patients must have access to these services and therapies as part of their comprehensive cancer care"[111]. As part of the Choosing Wisely initiative of the American Board of Internal Medicine, the American Academy of Hospice and Palliative Medicine states there should not be a delay in Palliative Care for any patients living with serious illness or in any distress due to disease directed treatment. As stated above, data shows that Palliative Medicine improves pain and symptom control, improves caregiver satisfaction with care and reduces healthcare costs [112]. These national recommendations mirror international statements. The Associazone Italiana di Oncologia Medica states that the mission of Medical Oncology should "follow the non-abandonment culture, guaranteeing quality of life and continuity of care to all cancer patients at every step of the disease, always considering the patient instead of the disease as the most important target"[113]. The European Society of Medical Oncology also emphasizes that Palliative Care should be "utilized whenever needs are identified, irrespective of stage of disease" not only at end-of-life [114].

5.1. Barriers

5.1.1. Workforce Shortages

An acute shortage of Palliative Medicine specialists exists. Rapid expansion of Palliative Care programs has occurred over the past 2-3 decades with the emergence of new data demonstrating the benefit of these programs in regards to improved patient care, cost of care and patient and family satisfaction. This has led to both nursing and physician shortages in the field of Palliative Medicine. The Center to Advance Palliative Care (CAPC) recommends a staffing ratio of at least one Palliative Care physician for every 250-350 inpatient hospital beds [115]. This level of staffing assumes not just one physician but a full interdisciplinary team including advance practice practitioners, nurses and social workers. Only 25% of hospital programs meet federally defined standards for having a complete Palliative Care team [116]. The Joint Commission's Advanced Certification Program for Palliative Care states that the team should include members with specialized training or experience in Palliative Care and must consist of a physician, a nurse which may include an advanced practice practitioner, a chaplain and a social worker [117]. Some data from academic Palliative Medicine centers has shown the use of at least one physician and physician assistant for every 155 beds. A 2009 study by the American Academy of Hospice and Palliative Medicine estimated the need for 6,000 to 18,000 individual Hospice and Palliative Medicine physicians to fulfill demands, with only 4,400 physicians available at the time of the study. The current capacity of fellowship programs is insufficient to resolve this lack of available physicians [118]. The current Hospice and Palliative Medicine workforce is unable to fulfill the needs of the quantity of oncology patients recommended for referral by national guidelines. Therefore, the importance of primary Palliative Care education for oncologists and all learners is essential as is the need for increased support and funding of Hospice and Palliative Medicine graduate medical education.

5.1.2. Lack of Palliative Care Understanding

Three main barriers expressed by Oncologists for Palliative Care referrals included the perception that Palliative Care is a philosophy incompatible with cancer treatment, the belief that providing this level of care is the role of the oncologist and lack of awareness of institutional or community services [119]. The greatest barrier to integration of Palliative Care into the treatment of patients with cancer may be the perception that it deals solely with the end-of-life [120]. The Medicare hospice benefit adds to this divide. This benefit provides hospice to patients with a prognosis of less than 6 months with the agreement to forgo treatments of curative or life prolonging intent. Hospice organizations are paid a daily rate for each patient, dis-incentivizing costly services to palliate or prevent patient symptoms that may be facilitated by Palliative Medicine services with regular cost coverage [121]. Cancer treatments may prolong survival as well as palliate cancer symptoms. For example radiation is often used to palliate symptoms of pain or tumor compression and yet Palliative Care is often depicted as care that happens when there is nothing left to offer [122]. Failure to recognize the scope of care within Palliative Medicine will result in patients with advanced cancer lacking maximum efforts at patient-centered, holistic care. A survey of American Oncologists and advanced practice providers indicated that 60% considered the term Palliative Care synonymous with end-of-life and hospice and was a barrier to referral by 23% of respondents [120].

Oncologists may believe they are providing their own effective Palliative Care. A survey of physicians in the Eastern Cooperative Oncology Group indicated that only half believed they were providing effective pain control to cancer patients and a third did not feel they should provide maximum pain control until patient prognosis was less than 6 months [123]. Another survey of oncologists in 2010 found that 87% recommended incorrect pain management recommendations when tested on clinical vignettes [124]. These studies support the need for improved clinician education regarding pain control, highlighting why pain is the most common symptom addressed by secondary and tertiary Palliative Medicine in Oncology.

Increased awareness and utilization of Palliative Care in Oncology will require education regarding the breadth of Palliative Medicine practice and the scope of services available by institution and location. An evaluation of German medical students in their final year of training found that less than 10% declared confidence in dealing with issues related to Palliative Care. This was similarly seen in the Netherlands where only 35% of medical students related their Palliative Care education as "good." A 2004 survey of hematology-oncology fellows in the United States found that more than half rated their Palliative Medicine education as poor [125-127]. Since 2013, Germany has mandated all medical students receive Palliative Medicine education as part of their curriculum and a push to develop disease-specific guidelines for timing of integration of Palliative Care into Oncology have developed [128, 129]. Efforts are being made for large scale Palliative Care education including the Education in Palliative and End of Life Care (EPEC) and Advocating for Clinical Excellence (ACE) programs to provide advocacy and increased knowledge of Palliative Care services [130-133].

6. Expert Opinion

Palliative Medicine has an important patient-centered role in Oncology practice from the time patients are diagnosed, through progression through outpatient and hospital based treatments and concluding with end-of-life care or survivorship. Oncologists and other physicians caring for serious illness are primary Palliative Care clinicians who are responsible for maximizing patient symptom control and quality of life during diagnosis and treatment. The responsibility to fulfill this role also includes the knowledge to know when the most beneficial time is to request Palliative Medicine consultation to avoid and relieve patient and caregiver distress. Patients with any serious illness deserve exceptional and early symptom management and supportive care. All Oncology patients warrant the setting and opportunity to consider and communicate their wishes for advanced care planning. Oncologists and Palliative Medicine clinicians can serve as close colleagues and strong patient advocates in the pursuit of these tasks. Effective collaboration with Palliative Medicine improves patient outcomes, is cost effective and has the broad support of clinical research and treatment guidelines. Barriers to Palliative Medicine include support of Palliative Care fellowships and educational programs as well as effective communication among clinicians to educate and clarify misconceptions of the roles Palliative Medicine can perform. Further research is needed to understand the gaps in effectively treating cancer symptoms and distress by primary Palliative Care clinicians such as Oncologists. Research is also needed in models of integration of Palliative Medicine into Oncology practice and the development of clinical pathways for patient referrals.

References

[1] *Center to Advance Palliative Care and National Palliative Care Research Cente*r. National Palliative Care Registry. August 15, 2016.; Available from: https://registry.capc.org/metrics-resources/summary-data/.

[2] Temel, J. S., et al., Early palliative care for patients with metastatic non-small-cell lung cancer. *N Engl J Med,* 2010. 363(8): p. 733-42.

[3] Holland, J. M., et al., Family evaluation of hospice care: Examining direct and indirect associations with overall satisfaction and caregiver confidence. *Palliat Support Car*e, 2015. 13(4): p. 901-8.

[4] Kim, S. H., et al., Association between the emotional status of family caregivers and length of stay in a palliative care unit: A retrospective study. *Palliat Support Care*, 2015. 13(6): p. 1695-700.

[5] Swarm, R., et al., Adult Cancer Pain. *Journal of the National Comprehensive Cancer Network*, 2010. 8(9): p. 1046-1086.

[6] Thompson, J. A., New NCCN Guidelines: Recognition and Management of Immunotherapy-Related Toxicity. *Journal of the National Comprehensive Cancer Network*, 2018. 16(5S): p. 594-596.

[7] Berger, M. J., et al., NCCN Guidelines Insights: Antiemesis, Version 2.2017. *Journal of the National Comprehensive Cancer Network,* 2017. 15(7): p. 883-893.

[8] Berger, A. M., et al., Cancer-Related Fatigue, Version 2.2015. *Journal of the National Comprehensive Cancer Network*, 2015. 13(8): p. 1012-1039.

[9] Distress Management Clinical Practice Guidelines in Oncology. *Journal of the National Comprehensive Cancer Network*, 2003. 1(3): p. 344.

[10] Hui, D., Definition of supportive care: does the semantic matter? *Current Opinion in Oncology*, 2014. 26(4): p. 372-9.

[11] Hui, D. and E. Bruera, Integrating palliative care into the trajectory of cancer care. *Nat Rev Clin Oncol,* 2016. 13(3): p. 159-71.

[12] Hannon, B., et al., Early Palliative Care and Its Role in Oncology: A Qualitative Study. *The Oncologist*, 2016. 21(11): p. 1387-1395.

[13] Dow, L. A., et al., Paradoxes in advance care planning: the complex relationship of oncology patients, their physicians, and advance medical directives. *J Clin Oncol,* 2010. 28(2): p. 299-304.

[14] Bakitas, M., et al., Effects of a palliative care intervention on clinical outcomes in patients with advanced cancer: the Project ENABLE II randomized controlled trial. *JAMA,* 2009. 302(7): p. 741-9.

[15] Bakitas, M., et al., Project ENABLE: a palliative care demonstration project for advanced cancer patients in three settings. *J Palliat Med,* 2004. 7(2): p. 363-72.

[16] von Gunten, C. F., Secondary and tertiary palliative care in us hospitals. *JAMA*, 2002. 287(7): p. 875-881.

[17] Hui, D., et al., Quality of end-of-life care in patients with hematologic malignancies: a retrospective cohort study. *Cancer,* 2014. 120(10): p. 1572-8.

[18] Howell, D. A., et al., Haematological malignancy: are patients appropriately referred for specialist palliative and hospice care? A systematic review and meta-analysis of published data. *Palliat Med,* 2011. 25(6): p. 630-41.

[19] Odejide, O. O., et al., Why are patients with blood cancers more likely to die without hospice? *Cancer,* 2017. 123(17): p. 3377-3384.

[20] Haun, M. W., et al., Early palliative care for adults with advanced cancer. *Cochrane Database of Systematic Revie*ws, 2017(6).

[21] Schwartzberg, L. S., et al., Chemotherapy-Induced Nausea and Vomiting (CINV) in Hematologic Malignancy Patients Receiving Multi-Day Highly Emetogenic Chemotherapy (HEC). *Blood,* 2016. 128(22): p. 2410.

[22] Gilmore, J. W., et al., Antiemetic Guideline Consistency and Incidence of Chemotherapy-Induced Nausea and Vomiting in US Community Oncology Practice: INSPIRE Study. *Journal of Oncology Practice,* 2014. 10(1): p. 68-74.

[23] Breuer, B., et al., How Well Do Medical Oncologists Manage Chronic Cancer Pain? A National Survey. *The Oncologist,* 2015. 20(2): p. 202-209.

[24] Selvaggi, K. J., et al., Bridging the gap: a palliative care consultation service in a hematological malignancy-bone marrow transplant unit. *J Community Support Oncol,* 2014. 12(2): p. 50-5.

[25] Rabow, M. W., et al., The comprehensive care team: a controlled trial of outpatient palliative medicine consultation. *Archives of internal medicine,* 2004. 164(1): p. 83-91.

[26] Bakitas, M., et al., Effects of a palliative care intervention on clinical outcomes in patients with advanced cancer: the Project ENABLE II randomized controlled trial. *JAMA,* 2009. 302(7): p. 741-749.

[27] Kostopoulou, S., et al., Advanced Cancer Patients' Perceptions of Dignity: The Impact of Psychologically Distressing Symptoms and Preparatory Grief. *Journal of Palliative Care*, 2018. 33(2): p. 88-94.

[28] E, K.-R., *On death and dying: what the dying have to teach doctors, nurses, clergy, and their families.* 1st edition ed. 1997, New York: Simon and Schuster.

[29] Caroff, S. N., et al., Recurrent idiopathic catatonia: implications beyond the diagnostic and statistical manual of mental disorders 5th edition. *Clinical Psychopharmacology and Neuroscience*, 2015. 13(2): p. 218.

[30] Boelen, P. A. and H. G. Prigerson, The influence of symptoms of prolonged grief disorder, depression, and anxiety on quality of life among bereaved adults. *European Archives of Psychiatry and Clinical Neuroscience*, 2007. 257(8): p. 444-452.

[31] Maciejewski, P. K., et al., An empirical examination of the stage theory of grief. *JAMA,* 2007. 297(7): p. 716-723.

[32] Prescott, A. T., et al., The role of a palliative care intervention in moderating the relationship between depression and survival among individuals with advanced cancer. *Health Psychol*, 2017. 36(12): p. 1140-1146.

[33] Nielsen, M. K., et al., Predictors of complicated grief and depression in bereaved caregivers: a nationwide prospective cohort study. *Journal of pain and symptom management,* 2017. 53(3): p. 540-550.

[34] Kuo, S.-C., et al., Longitudinal changes in and modifiable predictors of the prevalence of severe depressive symptoms for family caregivers of terminally ill cancer patients over the first two years of bereavement. *Journal of palliative medicine,* 2017. 20(1): p. 15-22.

[35] Puchalski, C., et al., Improving the Quality of Spiritual Care as a Dimension of Palliative Care: The Report of the Consensus Conference. *Journal of Palliative Medicine,* 2009. 12(10): p. 885-904.

[36] Balboni, T. A., et al., Provision of Spiritual Care to Patients With Advanced Cancer: Associations With Medical Care and Quality of Life Near Death. *Journal of Clinical Oncology,* 2010. 28(3): p. 445-452.

[37] Balducci, L., Geriatric Oncology, Spirituality, and Palliative Care. *J Pain Symptom Manage,* 2018.

[38] Vallurupalli, M., et al., The role of spirituality and religious coping in the quality of life of patients with advanced cancer receiving palliative radiation therapy. *The journal of supportive oncology,* 2012. 10(2): p. 81-87.

[39] Matos, T. D. d. S., et al., Quality of life and religious-spiritual coping in palliative cancer care patients. *Revista latino-americana de enfermagem,* 2017. 25: p. e2910-e2910.

[40] Murata, H., Spiritual pain and its care in patients with terminal cancer: construction of a conceptual framework by philosophical approach. *Palliat Support Care,* 2003. 1(1): p. 15-21.

[41] Delgado-Guay, M. O., et al., Spirituality, religiosity, and spiritual pain in advanced cancer patients. *J Pain Symptom Manage*, 2011. 41(6): p. 986-94.

[42] Delgado-Guay, M. O., et al., Frequency, intensity, and correlates of spiritual pain in advanced cancer patients assessed in a supportive/palliative care clinic. *Palliative and Supportive Care,* 2015. 14(4): p. 341-348.

[43] Hills, J., et al., Spirituality and Distress in Palliative Care Consultation. *Journal of Palliative Medicin*e, 2005. 8(4): p. 782-788.

[44] Katz, S., et al., Studies of illness in the aged: The index of adl: a standardized measure of biological and psychosocial function. *JAMA,* 1963. 185(12): p. 914-919.

[45] AARP. 2015 *Report Caregiving in the U.S.* 2015 3/28/2017]; Available from: http://www.caregiving.org.

[46] Deniz, H. and F. Inci, The burden of care and quality of life of caregivers of leukemia and lymphoma patients following peripheric stem cell transplantation. *J Psychosoc Oncol,* 2015. 33(3): p. 250-62.

[47] Nijboer, C., et al., The role of social and psychologic resources in caregiving of cancer patients. *Cancer,* 2001. 91(5): p. 1029-39.

[48] Kurtz, M. E., et al., Physical functioning and depression among older persons with cancer. *Cancer Pract*, 2001. 9(1): p. 11-8.

[49] Bevans, M. and E. M. Sternberg, Caregiving burden, stress, and health effects among family caregivers of adult cancer patients. *JAMA,* 2012. 307(4): p. 398-403.

[50] Nijboer, C., et al., Cancer and caregiving: the impact on the caregiver's health. *Psychooncology,* 1998. 7(1): p. 3-13.

[51] Beattie, S. and S. Lebel, The experience of caregivers of hematological cancer patients undergoing a hematopoietic stem cell transplant: a comprehensive literature review. *Psychooncology,* 2011. 20(11): p. 1137-50.

[52] Fife, B. L., et al., Adaptation of family caregivers during the acute phase of adult BMT. *Bone Marrow Transplant,* 2009. 43(12): p. 959-66.

[53] Boyle, D., et al., Caregiver quality of life after autologous bone marrow transplantation. *Cancer Nurs,* 2000. 23(3): p. 193-203; quiz 204-5.

[54] Dionne-Odom, J. N., et al., Benefits of Early Versus Delayed Palliative Care to Informal Family Caregivers of Patients With Advanced Cancer: Outcomes From the ENABLE III Randomized Controlled Trial. *J Clin Oncol,* 2015. 33(13): p. 1446-52.

[55] WHO Center for Development Ageing and health technical report Vol 5: *A glossary of terms for health care and services for older people.* 2004 [cited 2018; Available from: http://www.who.int/kobe_centre/ageing/ahp_vol5_glossary.pdf.

[56] Fine, R. L., From Quinlan to Schiavo: medical, ethical, and legal issues in severe brain injury. *Proceedings (Baylor University. Medical Center)*, 2005. 18(4): p. 303-310.

[57] Koch, K. A., Patient Self-Determination Act. *J Fla Med Assoc*, 1992. 79(4): p. 240-3.

[58] Garrido, M. M., et al., Quality of Life and Cost of Care at the End of Life: The Role of Advance Directives. *Journal of pain and symptom management,* 2015. 49(5): p. 828-835.

[59] Brinkman-Stoppelenburg, A., J. A. C. Rietjens, and A. van der Heide, The effects of advance care planning on end-of-life care: A systematic review. *Palliative Medicine*, 2014. 28(8): p. 1000-1025.

[60] McDonald, J. C., et al., Advance directives in patients with advanced cancer receiving active treatment: attitudes, prevalence, and barriers. *Supportive Care in Cancer,* 2017. 25(2): p. 523-531.

[61] Green, M. J., et al., Advance Care Planning Does Not Adversely Affect Hope or Anxiety Among Patients With Advanced Cancer. *J Pain Symptom Manage,* 2015. 49(6): p. 1088-96.

[62] Bakitas, M. A., et al., The TEAM Approach to Improving Oncology Outcomes by Incorporating Palliative Care in Practice. *Journal of Oncology Practice,* 2017. 13(9): p. 557-566.

[63] Ferrell, B. R., et al., Integration of Palliative Care Into Standard Oncology Care: ASCO Clinical Practice Guideline Update Summary. *J Oncol Pract,* 2017. 13(2): p. 119-121.

[64] Bruera, E. and D. Hui, Conceptual models for integrating palliative care at cancer centers. *J Palliat Med,* 2012. 15(11): p. 1261-9.

[65] Davis, M. P., F. Strasser, and N. Cherny, How well is palliative care integrated into cancer care? A MASCC, ESMO, and EAPC Project. *Support Care Cancer,* 2015. 23(9): p. 2677-85.

[66] Davis, M. P., et al., MASCC/ESMO/EAPC survey of palliative programs. *Support Care Cancer,* 2015. 23(7): p. 1951-68.

[67] Hui, D., et al., Improving patient and caregiver outcomes in oncology: Team-based, timely, and targeted palliative care. *CA: A Cancer Journal for Clinicians,* 2018. 68(5): p. 356-376.

[68] Coleman, E. A., Falling through the cracks: challenges and opportunities for improving transitional care for persons with continuous complex care needs. *J Am Geriatr Soc*, 2003. 51(4): p. 549-55.

[69] Muir, J. C., et al., Integrating palliative care into the outpatient, private practice oncology setting. *J Pain Symptom Manage*, 2010. 40(1): p. 126-35.

[70] Goldsmith, B., et al., Variability in access to hospital palliative care in the United States. *Journal of palliative medicine,* 2008. 11(8): p. 1094-1102.

[71] Smith, T. J., et al., A High-Volume Specialist Palliative Care Unit and Team May Reduce In-Hospital End-of-Life Care Costs. *Journal of Palliative Medicine*, 2003. 6(5): p. 699-705.

[72] Nathaniel, J. D., et al., Cost Savings Associated With an Inpatient Palliative Care Unit: Results from the First Two Years. *J Pain Symptom Manage,* 2015. 50(2): p. 147-54.

[73] Muir, J. C., et al., Integrating Palliative Care Into the Outpatient, Private Practice Oncology Setting. *Journal of Pain and Symptom Management,* 2010. 40(1): p. 126-135.

[74] Hui, D., et al., Impact of timing and setting of palliative care referral on quality of end-of-life care in cancer patients. *Cancer,* 2014. 120(11): p. 1743-1749.

[75] Scheffey, C., et al., Clinic-Based Outpatient Palliative Care Before Hospice Is Associated With Longer Hospice Length of Service. *Journal of Pain and Symptom Management,* 2014. 48(4): p. 532-539.

[76] Hui, D., et al., Referral Criteria for Outpatient Palliative Cancer Care: A Systematic Review. *The oncologist,* 2016. 21(7): p. 895-901.

[77] Cherny, N. I., Stigma associated with "palliative care": getting around it or getting over it. *Cancer,* 2009. 115(9): p. 1808-12.

[78] Roeland, E. and G. Ku, Spanning the canyon between stem cell transplantation and palliative care. *Hematology Am Soc Hematol Educ Program,* 2015. 2015: p. 484-9.

[79] Dalal, S., et al., Association between a name change from palliative to supportive care and the timing of patient referrals at a comprehensive cancer center. *Oncologist,* 2011. 16(1): p. 105-11.

[80] Fadul, N., et al., Supportive versus palliative care: what's in a name?: a survey of medical oncologists and midlevel providers at a comprehensive cancer center. *Cancer,* 2009. 115(9): p. 2013-21.

[81] Hui, D., et al., Attitudes and Beliefs toward Supportive and Palliative Care Referral among Hematologic and Solid Tumor Oncology Specialists. *Oncologist,* 2015. 20(11): p. 1326-32.

[82] Wentlandt, K., et al., Referral practices of oncologists to specialized palliative care. *J Clin Oncol,* 2012. 30(35): p. 4380-6.

[83] Maciasz, R. M., et al., Does it matter what you call it? A randomized trial of language used to describe palliative care services. *Support Care Cancer,* 2013. 21(12): p. 3411-9.

[84] Levy, M. H., et al., Palliative care. *J Natl Compr Canc Netw,* 2012. 10(10): p. 1284-309.

[85] Lee, S. J., et al., Routine screening for psychological distress on an Australian inpatient haematology and oncology ward: impact on use of psychosocial services. *Med J Aust,* 2010. 193(5 Suppl): p. S74-8.

[86] Wagner, L. I., et al., Bringing PROMIS to practice: brief and precise symptom screening in ambulatory cancer care. *Cancer,* 2015. 121(6): p. 927-34.

[87] Adelson, K., et al., Standardized Criteria for Palliative Care Consultation on a Solid Tumor Oncology Service Reduces Downstream Health Care Use. J*ournal of Oncology Practice*, 2017: p. JOP.2016.016808.

[88] Hui, D., et al., Availability and integration of palliative care at us cancer centers. *JAMA,* 2010. 303(11): p. 1054-1061.

[89] Cheng, W.-W., et al., Interval between Palliative Care Referral and Death among Patients Treated at a Comprehensive Cancer Center. *Journal of Palliative Medicine*, 2005. 8(5): p. 1025-1032.

[90] Morita, T., et al., Late Referrals to Palliative Care Units in Japan: Nationwide Follow-Up Survey and Effects of Palliative Care Team Involvement After the Cancer Control Act. *Journal of Pain and Symptom Management,* 2009. 38(2): p. 191-196.

[91] Hui, D., et al., Automatic referral to standardize palliative care access: an international Delphi survey. *Supportive Care in Cancer,* 2018. 26(1): p. 175-180.

[92] Glare, P. A., et al., Palliative care in the outpatient oncology setting: evaluation of a practical set of referral criteria. *Journal of oncology practice,* 2011. 7(6): p. 366-370.

[93] Atreya, S., Referral Patterns of Gynecological Cancer Patients to a Palliative Medicine Unit: A 2 Years Retrospective Analysis. *Indian journal of palliative care,* 2017. 23(4): p. 409-412.

[94] Wright, A. A., et al., Associations between end-of-life discussions, patient mental health, medical care near death, and caregiver bereavement adjustment. *JAMA,* 2008. 300(14): p. 1665-1673.

[95] Wong, A. K. Y., Referral patterns to palliative care: An inpatient snapshot study. *Journal of Clinical Oncology,* 2016. 34(26_suppl): p. 119-119.

[96] Hui, D., et al., Pattern and Predictors of Outpatient Palliative Care Referral Among Thoracic Medical Oncologists. *The Oncologist,* 2018. 23(10): p. 1230-1235.

[97] Rocque, G. B., et al., Inpatient hospitalization of oncology patients: are we missing an opportunity for end-of-life care? *J Oncol Pract,* 2013. 9(1): p. 51-4.

[98] Adelson, K., et al., Standardized Criteria for Palliative Care Consultation on a Solid Tumor Oncology Service Reduces Downstream Health Care Use. *J Oncol Pract,* 2017: p. JOP2016016808.

[99] May, P., et al., Palliative Care Teams' Cost-Saving Effect Is Larger For Cancer Patients with Higher Numbers of Comorbidities. *Health Aff* (Millwood), 2016. 35(1): p. 44-53.

[100] May, P., et al., Prospective Cohort Study of Hospital Palliative Care Teams for Inpatients With Advanced Cancer: Earlier Consultation Is Associated With Larger Cost-Saving Effect. *Journal of Clinical Oncology,* 2015. 33(25): p. 2745-2752.

[101] Starks, H., et al., Cost savings vary by length of stay for inpatients receiving palliative care consultation services. *J Palliat Med,* 2013. 16(10): p. 1215-20.

[102] McCarthy, I. M., et al., Cost savings from palliative care teams and guidance for a financially viable palliative care program. *Health Serv Res*, 2015. 50(1): p. 217-36.

[103] Morrison, R. S., et al., Palliative care consultation teams cut hospital costs for Medicaid beneficiaries. *Health Aff* (Millwood), 2011. 30(3): p. 454-63.

[104] Blackhall, L. J., et al., CARE Track for Advanced Cancer: Impact and Timing of an Outpatient Palliative Care Clinic. *Journal of Palliative Medicine*, 2016. 19(1): p. 57-63.

[105] Scibetta, C., et al., The Costs of Waiting: Implications of the Timing of Palliative Care Consultation among a Cohort of Decedents at a Comprehensive Cancer Center. *J Palliat Med,* 2016. 19(1): p. 69-75.

[106] Centers for Medicare and Medicaid Services. *Proposed policy, payment, and quality provisions changes to the Medicare Physician Fee Schedule for Calendar Year 2017.* June 13, 2017]; Available from: www.cms.gov/Newsroom/MediaReleaseDatabase/Factsheets/2017-Fact-sheets.html.

[107] Cowan, J. D., Hospital charges for a community inpatient palliative care program. *Am J Hosp Palliat Care,* 2004. 21(3): p. 177-90.

[108] Ciemins, E. L., et al., The economic and clinical impact of an inpatient palliative care consultation service: a multifaceted approach. *J Palliat Med*, 2007. 10(6): p. 1347-55.

[109] Ferrell, B. R., et al., Integration of Palliative Care Into Standard Oncology Care: American Society of Clinical Oncology Clinical Practice Guideline Update. *J Clin Oncol,* 2017. 35(1): p. 96-112.

[110] Landrum, L. M., et al., Comprehensive care in gynecologic oncology: The importance of palliative care. *Gynecol Oncol,* 2015. 137(2): p. 193-202.

[111] Edwards, M. J., Access to quality cancer care: consensus statement of the American Federation of Clinical Oncologic Societies. *Annals of surgical oncology*, 1998. 5(7): p. 657-659.

[112] Fischberg, D., et al., Five things physicians and patients should question in hospice and palliative medicine. *J Pain Symptom Manage,* 2013. 45(3): p. 595-605.

[113] Zagonel, V., et al., The Medical Oncologist's Role in Palliative Care: AIOM's Position. *Tumori Journal,* 2009. 95(6): p. 652-654.

[114] Cherny, N., et al., European Society for Medical Oncology (ESMO) Program for the Integration of Oncology and Palliative Care: a 5-year review of the Designated Centers' incentive program. *Annals of Oncology*, 2010. 21(2): p. 362-369.

[115] Ahluwalia, S. C., et al., A Systematic Review in Support of the National Consensus Project Clinical Practice Guidelines for Quality

Palliative Care, Fourth Edition. *Journal of Pain and Symptom Management.*

[116] Spetz, J., et al., Few Hospital Palliative Care Programs Meet National Staffing Recommendations. *Health Affairs,* 2016. 35(9): p. 1690-1697.

[117] Weissman, D. E. and D. E. Meier, Operational features for hospital palliative care programs: consensus recommendations. *Journal of palliative medicine*, 2008. 11(9): p. 1189-1194.

[118] Lupu, D., Estimate of Current Hospice and Palliative Medicine Physician Workforce Shortage. *Journal of Pain and Symptom Management,* 2010. 40(6): p. 899-911.

[119] Schenker, Y., et al., Oncologist Factors That Influence Referrals to Subspecialty Palliative Care Clinics. *Journal of Oncology Practice,* 2014. 10(2): p. e37-e44.

[120] Von Roenn, J. H., R. Voltz, and A. Serrie, Barriers and Approaches to the Successful Integration of Palliative Care and Oncology Practice. *Journal of the National Comprehensive Cancer Network,* 2013. 11(suppl 1): p. S-11-S-16.

[121] Malin, J. L., Bridging the Divide: Integrating Cancer-Directed Therapy and Palliative Care. *Journal of Clinical Oncology*, 2004. 22(17): p. 3438-3440.

[122] Detmar, S. B., et al., Role of Health-Related Quality of Life in Palliative Chemotherapy Treatment Decisions. *Journal of Clinical Oncology,* 2002. 20(4): p. 1056-1062.

[123] Von Roenn, J. H., et al., Physician attitudes and practice in cancer pain management: A survey from the eastern cooperative oncology group. *Annals of Internal Medicine,* 1993. 119(2): p. 121-126.

[124] Breuer, B., et al., Medical Oncologists' Attitudes and Practice in Cancer Pain Management: A National Survey. *Journal of Clinical Oncology,* 2011. 29(36): p. 4769-4775.

[125] Weber, M., et al., Knowledge and attitude of final - year medical students in Germany towards palliative care - an interinstitutional questionnaire-based study. *BMC Palliative Care*, 2011. 10(1): p. 19.

[126] Hesselink, B. A. M., et al., Education on End-of-Life Care in the Medical Curriculum: Students' Opinions and Knowledge. *Journal of Palliative Medicine*, 2010. 13(4): p. 381-387.

[127] Buss, M. K., et al., A study of oncology fellows' training in end-of-life care. *The journal of supportive oncology,* 2007. 5(5): p. 237-242.

[128] Alt-Epping, B., et al., Implementing the cross-disciplinary subject of palliative medicine (Q13) against the backdrop of recent changes of the legal framework using University Medical School Göttingen as an example. *GMS Zeitschrift für medizinische Ausbildung*, 2010. 27(5).

[129] Gaertner, J., et al., Standardizing integration of palliative care into comprehensive cancer therapy—a disease specific approach. *Supportive Care in Cancer*, 2011. 19(7): p. 1037.

[130] Emanuel, L., et al., *The education in palliative and end-of-life care (EPEC) curriculum.* Chicago: The EPEC Project, 2003.

[131] Robinson, K., et al., Assessment of the education for physicians on end-of-life care (EPEC™) project. *Journal of palliative medicine,* 2004. **7**(5): p. 637-645.

[132] Emanuel, L., et al., EPEC-O: Education in Palliative and End-of-life Care for Oncology. *Module,* 2005. 2: p. 12-14.

[133] Otis-Green, S., et al., An overview of the ACE Project—advocating for clinical excellence: transdisciplinary palliative care education. *Journal of Cancer Education*, 2009. 24(2): p. 120-126.

In: New Developments in Oncology Research
Editor: Marcos T. Blair
ISBN: 978-1-53615-365-1
© 2019 Nova Science Publishers, Inc.

Chapter 2

ELECTROLYTE DISORDERS IN CANCER PATIENTS: CLINICAL IMPLICATION AND MANAGEMENT

Rossana Berardi*, Francesca Morgese, Silvia Rinaldi and Mariangela Torniai

Clinica Oncologica, Università Politecnica delle Marche,
Azienda Ospedaliero-Universitaria Ospedali Riuniti
Umberto I – GM Lancisi – G Salesi - Ancona, Italy

ABSTRACT

Electrolyte disorders are common in cancer patients and can determine a worsening prognosis. However, these alterations are often misunderstood or not considered in clinical practice. The most common electrolyte alterations involve sodium, potassium, calcium and magnesium serum level. These electrolyte disorders might be related either to cancer physiopathology (e.g., paraneoplastic syndromes such as the syndrome of

* Corresponding Author's Email: r.berardi@univpm.it.

inappropriate secretion of ADH-SIADH, tumor lysis syndrome, etc.), or anti-cancer agents or other concomitant treatments. Moreover, they are often multifactorial or can result from comorbidities or unknown causes.

Electrolyte disorders might cause life-threatening morbidity causing multiple organ systems dysfunction. Furthermore, emerging data showed that they might influence cancer patients' outcome, whether not promptly corrected. In particular, they seem to be correlated with poorer performance status, they might cause delays in therapy and negatively affect treatments' response and survival.

Therefore, it is necessary to better understand the physiological principles underlying these disorders and at the same time to achieve an early identification, in order to attempt an adequate and effective therapy and an appropriate monitoring.

This systematic review aims to better explain the mechanisms that underlie electrolyte disturbances in cancer patients, to stress on the serious prognostic implications involved and to provide practical and useful indications for the prompt diagnosis, management and therapy of electrolyte disorders.

Keywords: cancer, electrolyte disorders, hyponatremia, prognosis, electrolyte management

INTRODUCTION

Cancer patients often develop electrolyte disorders that may cause worsening prognosis. The most frequent electrolyte disorders involve altered serum levels of sodium, calcium, potassium and magnesium. These disorders may be caused by cancer metabolism, anti-tumor therapy or other concomitant medical conditions or treatments. Moreover, they may result from comorbidities or unknown causes, giving often important morbidity and being sometimes life threatening. They are often multifactorial and they might be both due to and responsible for dysfunction of multiple organ systems. Furthermore, they are often associated with worsening quality of life and prognosis, with a lower probability of tumor response to anti-cancer therapies and with delays in treatment schedule determining a negative impact in patients' outcome [1].

An ever-increasing attention towards electrolyte disturbances is emerging in the literature. A recent retrospective review of phase I studies carried out between 2011 and 2015 showed that most of the studies included data of electrolyte alterations (EAs) within toxicities. It demonstrated that hyponatraemia occurred in 62% of patients, hypokalemia in 40%, hypophosphatemia in 32%, hypomagnesaemia in 17% and hypocalcemia in 12%, and that diarrhea was associated with hypomagnesaemia at all grades ($p < 0.001$), hyponatraemia at all grades ($p = 0.006$) and with G3/G4 hypokalemia ($p = 0.02$). Furthermore, hyponatraemia was associated with a higher risk of developing other EAs during the trial in the univariate analysis [2].

Therefore, an early detection of electrolyte disorders and their prompt correction are crucial. Effective treatment depends on early identification, on understanding of physiological principles underlying the disorder, on attempt of adequate therapy to correct the disorder and on appropriate monitoring [1]. This manuscript aims i) to improve the knowledge on electrolyte disorders in cancer patients, underlying their prognostic impact whether not recognized and ii) to supply practical and useful indications for their prompt diagnosis and therapy in order to improve the management of these alterations.

METHODS

We extensively reviewed all available scientific literature regarding electrolytic alterations in cancer patients. MEDLINE, PUBMED and CancerLit databases were used in order to search studies published between 1982 and October 2018 on altered sodium, potassium, magnesium, phosphate and calcium serum balance. We restricted the research to publications in English and the research keywords included: sodium, potassium, magnesium, phosphate, calcium, chemotherapy, target therapies, immunotherapy, survival, and outcome, in association with cancer. Full articles were screened and additional appropriate references were checked.

In case of multiple publications concerning similar results, we selected and reported only the most recent one.

Sodium

Sodium is the primary extracellular constituent of serum osmolality. Its presence in the extracellular fluid (ECF) is critical to maintain circulating blood volume. Normally, about 25% of ECF is in the intravascular compartment and the remaining 75% in the interstitium.

The ECF represents about 1/3 of the total body water, distributed in the intracellular compartment (ICF), for the remaining and prevalent portion. Water and sodium concentrations are therefore strictly interdependent.

Sodium concentration is within a physiologic range of 135–145 mmol/l despite great variations in water and salt intake.

Normonatremia is maintained by an integrated system involving regulated water intake by thirst and control of water excretion by antidiuretic hormone secretion.

Changes in ECF and osmolality induce compensatory mechanisms involving modifications in renal sodium excretion and in renal free water clearance.

Renal sodium excretion is regulated by several mechanisms including glomerular filtration rate, adrenal aldosterone secretion and intrarenal hemodynamic and peritubular factors.

Furthermore angiotensin II, arginine vasopressin (AVP), atrial natriuretic peptide (ANP), dopamine, renal sympathetic nerve activity and renal prostaglandins may also influence renal sodium excretion [3-5].

The major determinant of serum sodium is serum water content, therefore sodium balance is closely related to water metabolism which is predominantly regulated by AVP and strongly influenced by water intake and output. AVP secretion in association to thirst maintains serum osmolality within a range that averages 285 mOsm/kg [6-11].

Abnormalities in water balance include hyponatremia and hypernatremia.

Hyponatremia

A serum sodium level below 135 mmol/l commonly defines hyponatremia.

According to its severity, it can be divided into three levels: mild (130-134 mEq/L), moderate (125-129 mEq/L) and severe (<125 mEq/L) [12-13]. According to time of onset it can be classified in acute (onset < 24 h) or chronic hyponatremia (onset > 24 h).

It is the most common electrolyte disorder linked to tumor-related conditions. However, its incidence is still unclear because of differences in cancer type, clinical setting, and serum sodium cut-off point.

Recent data have reported a variable incidence from 4% to 44% [14]. The most common neoplasm associated with hyponatraemia is small cell lung cancer (SCLC), with an incidence estimated around 15% [14].

Risk factors for hyponatremia include chemotherapy or its toxicity, fluids, also given with chemotherapy and opioids. Moreover, nausea can promote the release of AVP and vomiting also brings to gastrointestinal loss of sodium.

Focus on Hyponatremia in Cancer Patients

The incidence and prevalence of hyponatremia in cancer patients vary greatly, depending on the cancer type, clinical setting, and serum sodium cut-off point. Although only a few studies have evaluated the impact of hyponatremia on prognosis, it seems to be associated with a poor outcome [15]. In fact, it negatively influences performance status [16] and it has been reported to be a negative prognostic factor in cancer patients, especially in patients with lung cancer, [17], pleural mesothelioma [18], renal cell carcinoma [19], gastrointestinal cancer [20-21] and lymphoma [22]. Hyponatremia seems also to be an important negative predictive factor both for chemotherapy and for targeted therapy [23]. We previously demonstrated that hyponatremia have negative effects on hospitalization length and costs and on quality of life in cancer patients [24].

Some authors investigated the role of hyponatremia correction on patients' outcome, showing that those who reached sodium normalization had a better prognosis [25].

Symptoms

Hyponatremia is characterized by reduced serum sodium concentration; therefore, there is an osmotic shift of water from the ECF to ICF. The immediate consequence of this is cytoplasmic swelling. Symptoms depend on grade of hyponatremia and on onset speed (Table 1).

In case of mild hyponatremia (125 - 135 mEq/L) symptoms are commonly mild, vague, or completely absent. Patient often complain gastrointestinal symptoms, especially nausea and vomiting. At lower sodium concentrations, neurological symptoms predominate. In severe cases, hyponatremia can induce coma, respiratory depression and death. Moreover, greater is the speed of onset, greater is the number and severity of the symptoms. However, even the most nuanced symptoms of chronic hyponatraemia should not be underestimated because they are associated with an increased risk of falls, bone fractures and osteoporosis, complicating the already fragile condition of cancer patients [1].

Table 1. Hyponatremia symptoms

Na > 125 mEq/L	110 > Na >125 mEq/L	Na < 110 mEq/L
• Symptomless or blurred symptoms: • dizziness • postural instability • asthenia	Appetite loss, nausea, vomiting headache, irritability, altered mood, attention deficit, confusion disorientation, dizziness, gait disturbances, recurrent falls, bone fragility with reduced bone mineralization, muscle cramps, lethargy	Intense asthenia, drowsiness, reflex depression, bulbar paralysis, convulsions, encephalic brain herniation, coma, cardio-respiratory arrest

Causes

Hyponatremia can be classified, on the basis of the ECV status, in (Table 2):

- hypovolaemic, when ECV is reduced
- euvolaemic, when ECV is normal
- hypervolaemic, when ECV is increased.

Several conditions can contribute to hypovolemic hyponatremia such as vomiting, diarrhea, bleeding, renal fluid and solute losses and cerebral salt wasting (CSW), which is a hypothalamic-renal axis dysfunction characterized by natriuresis, volume depletion and subsequent AVP induced water retention.

Table 2. Hyponatremia causes

Extracellular volume (ECV)	Causes of hyponatremia
Ipovolemic	• Gastrointestinal losses (vomiting, diarrhea) • M. Addison • Diuretics • Neuropathies • Cerebral salt wasting syndrome
Euvolemic	• SIAD • Hypercortisolism • Hypothyroidism
Hypervolemic	• Cirrhosis • Heart failure • Kidney failure • Nephrotic syndrome

Syndrome of inappropriate antidiuresis (SIAD) is the main cause of hyponatremia in hospitalized patients and in cancer patients, affecting 1 to 2% of all patients and representing 30% of hyponatremia's cause in this setting [14]. SIAD is most frequently reported in SCLC but it is also common in non-small cell lung cancer, head and neck and breast cancer patients, while it is less frequent in other types of malignancies [14]. The term SIAD was proposed to replace syndrome from inappropriate secretion of ADH (SIADH) after the identification of cases with the clinical features of SIADH, but with ADH undetectable. In these patients an activating mutation of the ADH receptor V2 was identified [26-28].

Table 3. SIAD's causes

Tumors	– Pulmonary/mediastinal tumors (e.g., bronchogenic carcinoma, mesothelioma, thymic tumors) – Other neoplasms (duodenal, pancreatic, urothelial, nasopharyngeal, prostatic, uterine carcinoma and leukemia)
CNS diseases	– Expansive lesions (e.g., tumors, brain abscesses, subdural hematoma) – Inflammatory diseases (e.g., encephalitis, meningitis, systemic lupus, intermittent acute porphyria, multiple sclerosis) – Degenerative/demyelinating diseases (e.g., Guillain-Barré syndrome, spinal injuries) – Miscellaneous (e.g., subarachnoid hemorrhage, head injury, acute psychosis, delirium tremens, hypophyseal peduncle section, transphenoidal adenectomy, hydrocephalus).
Drug-induced (Table 4)	– Through the stimulation of the AVP release – Through strengthening the effect of AVP – Mixed or uncertain mechanism of action
Pulmonary diseases	– Infections (e.g., tuberculosis, acute bacterial or viral pneumonia, aspergillosis, empyema) – Mechanical/ventilator (e.g., respiratory failure, COPD, active pressure ventilation)
Others	– AIDS – Intense and prolonged physical exercise – Senile atrophy – Idiopathic

However, it is characterized by an inappropriate or persistent release of AVP that causes a decreased capacity free water excretion, which leads to serum hypo-osmolality and hyponatremia. [29]. In other cancers, hyponatraemia and in some cases SIAD are more frequently caused by pharmacological treatments (analgesics, chemotherapeutic agents, antidepressants, diuretics, antiemetics). Finally, drugs (such as chemotherapeutic treatments or targeted therapies) might induce hyponatraemia due to gastrointestinal side effects, including in particular vomiting and diarrhea [30].

There are several conditions that can lead to SIADH, such the central nervous system disorders, pulmonary disorders, medications and a variety of other causes (Table 3) [31].

SIADH may also result from ectopic production of AVP and ANP by the tumor tissue. It has also been associated with cytotoxic treatments including vinca alkoids, cisplatin, cyclophosphamide and melphalan (Table 4) [32]. We previously demonstrated, with a metanalysis, that also new biological drugs (in particular antiangiogenetic agent) increase the risk of hyponatremia [33].

Hypervolemic hyponatremia occurs in the context of an excess of total body water and sodium, which can be caused by cirrhosis, chronic kidney disease, congestive heart failure and manifested in edematous states [34-36].

According to serum osmolality, hyponatremia can also be classified as hypo-osmolar, iso-osmolar or hyper-osmolar.

Hyponatremia can be subdivided into:

- hypotonic (reduced serum osmolality)
- not hypotonic
- hypertonic (increased serum osmolality, as in glycemic decompensation);
- isotonic (normal serum osmolality, e.g., by absorption of sodium-free irrigating solutions used during uro/gynecological interventions).

Hypotonic hyponatremia can be hypovolemic, isovolemic or hypervolemic and may be frequently observed in several pathological conditions such as renal and endocrine disorders, SIADH, diuretic use, gastrointestinal sodium loss, cirrhosis, CHF, psychiatric illness or in infiltrative diseases of the hypothalamus. It is an expression of an excess of water compared to the sodium content that can be normal, increased or decreased.

Table 4. Main causes and mechanisms of drug-induced hyponatremia

Drugs with action on *sodium and water homeostasis*	Diuretics	Thiazide, indapamide, amiloride, loop diuretics
Drugs with action on water homeostasis: *Increased production of ADH*	Antidepressants Antipsychotics Antiepileptics Antitumor	Tricyclic (e.g., amitriptyline, protriptyline, desipramine), inhibitors of serotonin reuptake, monoamine oxidase inhibitors) Phenothiazines, haloperidol Carbamazepine, oxcarbazepine, sodium valproate Vinca alkaloids (vincristine and vinblastine) Platinum derivatives (cisplatin, carboplatin) Alkylating agents (cyclophosphamide, melphalan, ifosfamide) Miscellaneous (methotrexate, interferon, levamisole, pentostatin, monoclonal antibodies, target therapies) Opioids
Drugs with action on water homeostasis: *strengthening effect of ADH*	Antidiabetics Antiepileptics Antitumor NSAIDs	Chlorpropamide, tolbutamide Carbamazepine, lamotrigine Alkylating agents (cyclophosphamide e.v.)
Reset homeostat	Antidepressants Antiepileptics	Venlafaxine Carbamazepine

Excess water can be due to:

1. Excessive water intake with normal excretory capacity (e.g., primary polydipsia);
2. Altered renal water excretory capacity [37-38].

Iso-osmolar hyponatremia can occur when there is a reduction in the serum sodium and a storage of isotonic fluid to the ECF or in the presence of high levels of several compounds such as proteins and lipids in serum, not changing serum osmolality but resulting in an artificially hyponatremia (pseudohyponatremia) [39-41].

Diagnosis

Hyponatremia may be identified by routine laboratory testing or it can be suspected in the presence of neurological symptoms.

Symptoms related to hyponatremia are primarily due to cerebral edema and correlate both with the severity and with the rate of decline in serum sodium: they can vary from non-specific headache and mental impairment to confusion, nausea and vomit and, finally, to coma. Nevertheless, most patients may remain asymptomatic.

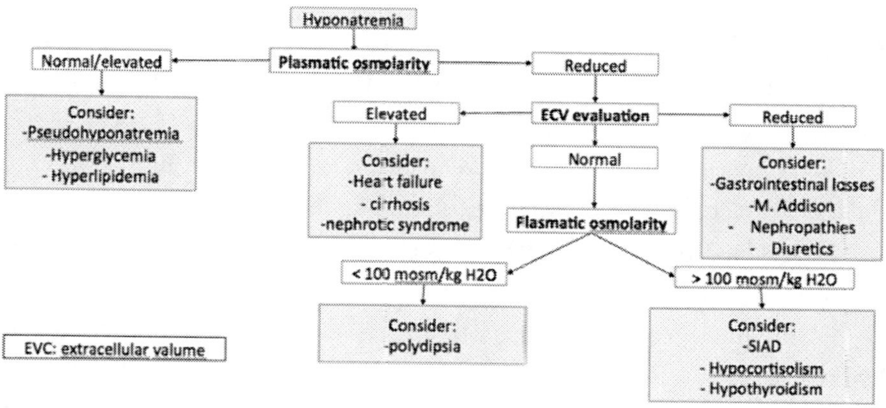

Figure 1. Diagnostic algorithm for hyponatremia.

Differential diagnosis of hyponatremia is based on clinical and laboratory assessment including plasma osmolality, urine osmolality, extracellular fluid volume status and urinary sodium levels [42]. Understanding the nature of hyponatraemia, is also crucial for a proper treatment approach (Figure 1).

SIAD is defined as a diagnosis of exclusion and the criteria are resumed in Table 5 [43-45]:

Table 5. SIAD diagnosis

Major criteria	Minor criteria
– Evidence of hyponatremia (<135 mEq/L) – Normal extracellular volume, – Serum hypo-osmolality (<275 mOsm/kg), – Inappropriately urine osmolality (above 100 mOsm/kg), – Urine sodium concentration >30 mmol/l, – Normal renal function, – Normal adrenal and thyroid function, – No use of diuretics.	– Plasmatic acid uric < 4 mg/dl – Blood urea nitrogen (BUN) > 10 mg/dl – Fractional sodium excretion > 1% – Fractional urea excretion > 55%

Treatment

Acting effectively and timely on the normalization of sodium levels could have a positive effect on prognosis of cancer patients [42] (Figure 2).

Treatment options include: fluid restriction, sodium administration, or the use of selective vasopressin receptor antagonists.

However, fluid restriction takes several days to correct serum sodium levels and it is frequently associated with poor patient compliance.

Furthermore, cancer patients often receive drugs that require abundant hydration.

Isotonic saline infusion may be used in states of volume depletion to correct hyponatremia.

The rate of correction should not exceed 12 mmol/liter/24 hours since an excessively rapid correction of hyponatremia can predispose to the development of cerebral oedema, central pontine myelinolysis, coma and death. To keep the correction speed under control, it is important to monitor the natremia at regular intervals, at least once every 4-6 hours.

When severe neurological symptoms are present, serum sodium may need to be corrected more rapidly.

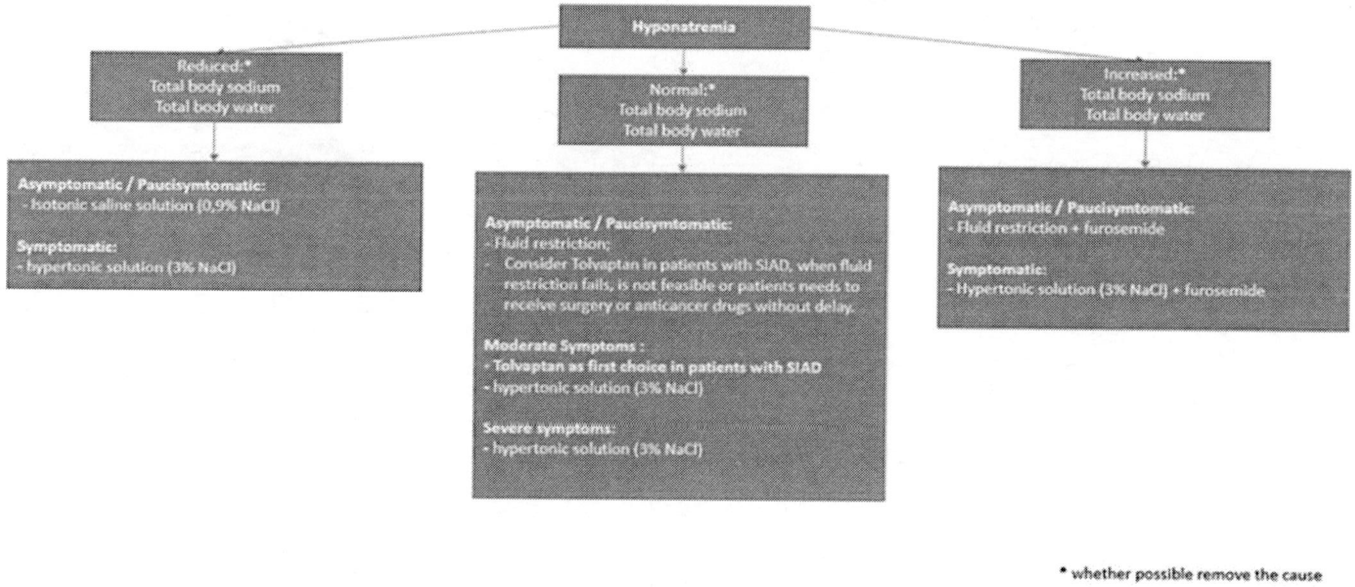

Figure 2. Hyponatremia treatment algorithm.

Administering 3% hypertonic saline represents an appropriate therapy for severe cases of hyponatremia also to increase free water excretion by the kidneys [42].

A new treatment of hyponatremia is represented by AVP-receptor antagonists, which are selective for the V2 receptor in the renal collecting ducts. They produce a selective water diuresis without affecting sodium and potassium excretion. Tolvaptan is approved in Europe for the treatment of hyponatremia secondary to SIAD. For an optimal management of patients, Tolvaptan therapy should be started in a hospital setting to check the therapeutic response. The starting dose is 15 mg once daily and it may be increased at 24 –hour intervals to a maximum of 60 mg once daily [46].

In a prospective study enrolling patients affected by SCLC with SIAD, tolvaptan demonstrated to correct and subsequently stabilize serum sodium levels, allowing them to receive chemotherapy without delay. Furthermore, tolvaptan reduces the risk of hyponatremia resulting from the same chemotherapy [47-49].

Other therapeutic options that can be used only in some Countries are urea and Demeclocycline. However, they are poorly used in clinical practice due to their poor tolerability.

The duration of treatment for hyponatraemia depends largely on the cause. In drug-induced hyponatraemia, electrolyte disturbance is usually restored within a few days of cessation of the drug involved. In contrast, in tumors that secrete ADH, hyponatraemia usually requires a longer and more unpredictable therapy, which also depends on the response to anti-cancer treatments [40]. Hyponatraemia should therefore be carefully considered and corrected in cancer patients, preferably avoiding severe restrictions on liquids or drugs that may increase nausea (urea), taking into account that serum sodium levels normalization has been positively correlated with the prognosis and with a reduction of length of hospital stay.

Hypernatremia

Hypernatremia is defined as a serum sodium concentration above 145 mmol/l.

It is a common electrolyte disorder affecting between 1% and 5% of hospitalized patients and it is associated with a significant high mortality (40-75%) when severe.

The reported prevalence of hypernatremia in non-critically ill hospitalized patients is of 0.2% before admission; a further 1% of patients develops hypernatremia during hospitalization [50].

Mortality rates in hypernatremic patients were reported to be dramatically increased as compared with normonatremic patients [51].

Symptoms

The clinical manifestations of hypernatremia are mainly neurological and correlate with both severity and onset speed: symptoms are more evident in case of a rapid increase of serum sodium level.

Initial symptoms are often non-specific:

- anorexia
- restlessness
- nausea
- muscle weakness
- lethargy
- intense thirst (usually extinguished by persistent hypernatremia)
- confusion
- These symptoms can progress to a more severe dysfunction of the central nervous system, which can lead to:
- hyperreflexia
- convulsions
- coma (in particular in the case of rapid sodium loading)

Brain dehydration induced by hypernatremia may cause complications such as cerebral/subarachnoid hemorrhage, with possible permanent damage or death [52].

Causes

The most common causes of hypernatraemia can be divided as follows (Table 6):

- those primarily due to a loss of free water
- those primarily caused by a positive sodium balance or a combination of both.

The loss of total body water is the commonest cause and it may be related to impaired thirst, reduced access to water, defected AVP release or AVP responsiveness.

Several factors have been associated with an increased risk of hypernatremia, including altered mental status, older age, prior brain injury or surgery, diuretic therapy and diabetes [53-54].

Thirst is the major defense against the onset of hypernatremia: in fact, it frequently develops when there is no access to free water as a consequence of impaired or altered sensation of thirst or neurologic injury with alterations to mental status. True deficits in thirst and osmoregulation are frequently described in patients with hypothalamic structural lesions caused by tumors, traumatic brain injury and vascular disease [55].

Water loss can be caused by either renal or extrarenal mechanism [56].

Renal water loss can be due to osmotic diuresis (i.e., hyperglycaemia, use of mannitol, increased serum urea concentration or administration of other hypertonic therapies) and to the use of diuretics [57].

Water diuresis can also be caused by insipidus diabetes, which is further divided into central and nephrogenic. Central insipidus diabetes is associated with a reduced secretion of AVP and it is frequently observed in cases of central nervous system damage or surgery (i.e., pituitary or hypothalamus malignancies and surgery or cranial irradiation) [58].

Nephrogenic insipidus diabetes results from renal resistance to the effects of AVP. Causes include inherited and acquired forms: the effects of ifosfamide or streptozocin on tubular reabsorption of water may induce nephrogenic diabetes insipidus although the cellular mechanism is not clearly understood [59-60].

Table 6. Causes of hypernatremia

Loss of free water	*Euvolemic:* - Losses through skin and breath - Reduced thirst stimulation - Neurogenic or nephrogenic diabetes insipidus *Hypovolemic:* - Renal causes (loop diuretics, osmotic diuresis, post-obstructive diuresis, acute tubular necrosis) - Gastro-intestinal causes (e.g., vomiting, nasogastric drainage, entero-cutaneous fistulae, diarrhea) - Cutaneous cause (burns, excessive sweating)
Sodium accumulation	- Hypertonic sodium bicarbonate infusion - Ingestion of NaCL/ingestion of marine H2O - Emetics rich in NaCl - Enema with hypertonic saline - Intra-uterine injection of hypertonic saline - Hypertonic dialysis - Primitive hyperaldosteronism - Cushing Syndrome

Further drugs, such as amphotericin B, lithium, ifosfamide and foscarnet, can be associated with nephrogenic insipidus diabetes [61-62].

Potential causes of extra-renal water loss include fluid losses from the gastrointestinal tract which can occur from vomiting, nasogastric drainage or diarrhoea. Acute and often severe hypernatremia can be induced by administering hypertonic solutions containing sodium or by ingesting a massive amount of salt.

Enteral nutrition with hyperosmolar or high protein feeds accompanied by insufficient free water may lead to hypernatremia, particularly in patients receiving chronic nutritional support [56].

Diagnosis

The initial step in managing of hypernatremia is confirming the diagnosis and discontinuing cause-specific predisposing factors (Figure 3).

In case of suspected neurological symptoms associated to thirst, the presence of hypernatremia should be considered.

Nevertheless, chronic hypernatraemia is much less likely to induce neurological symptoms thanks to the cerebral adaptation response that promptly restores cell volume and intense thirst may be absent, especially in patients with altered mental status or with hypothalamic lesions affecting the thirst center [63].

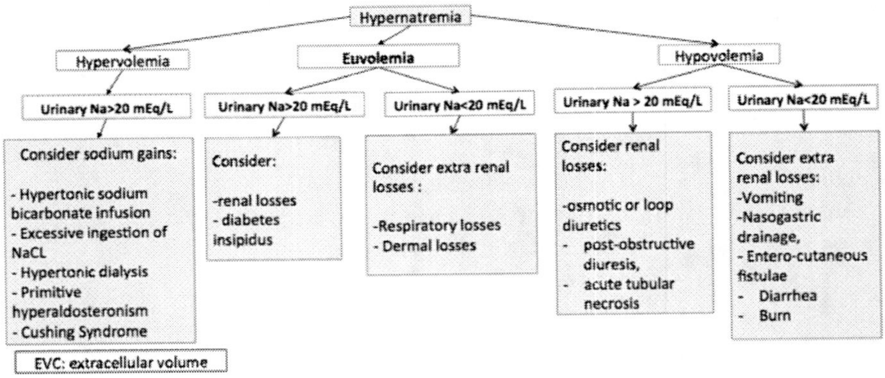

Figure 3. Diagnostic algorithm of hypernatremia.

Furthermore, it should be determined if hyponatremia is due to gain of sodium or loss of free water or whether a combination of the two causes is present.

It can usually be differentiated through the assessment of urine osmolality, urine sodium concentration and urine volume. The measurement of urinary sodium may be useful in differentiating a water loss from sodium overload [64].

Hypernatraemia should therefore be considered primarily a disorder of water balance.

When associated to concentrated urine, hypernatremia generally suggests insufficient water intake or gastrointestinal losses or sodium overload.

Conversely, a serum sodium >145 mmol/l or serum osmolality>295 mOsm/kg H2O associated with a urine osmolality <700–800 mOsm /kg H2O suggests a defect in urinary concentration [64].

The criteria for central insipidus diabetes diagnosis include polyuria (i.e., 24 hours urine volume exceeding 2.5 L) and high serum sodium levels. In the absence of causes of high urine osmolality this generally suggests the presence of insipidus diabetes [65].

Treatment

The management of hypernatremia consists in confirming diagnosis and then:

1. in removing the cause, where possible.
2. in correcting the hypernatremia (water deficit) based on the volemia with the restoration of intravascular volume and free water.

Oral hydration is effective in collaborating patients and in the absence of gastrointestinal dysfunction. In case of severe hypernatremia or in patients with difficulty in oral fluid intake due to vomiting or neurological changes, hydration e.v. represents a valid alternative.

When hypernatraemia develops in a short period (within 24 hours) or it is severely symptomatic, immediate treatment with isotonic solutions or hypotonic fluids should be started since a quick correction (up to 8-12 mmol/L per days) could improve the prognosis with no risk of convulsions and cerebral oedema. A correction of 1 mEq/L/h is considered safe in these patients [66, 67].

When hypernatraemia is chronic or with unknown temporal onset, it should be corrected within 48 hours, and serum osmolality should be reduced to a rate no higher than 0.5 mOsm/L/h to avoid the onset of cerebral edema. It is safe to reduce the serum sodium concentration slowly (8 to 10 mmol/L per day); moreover, treatment should be directed to the underlying cause. To keep the correction speed under control, natremia should be monitored at regular intervals, at least once every 4 hours [64].

If a loss of free water alone is present, it should be treated by the administration of free water (5% dextrose solution). In presence of pure sodium gain natriuresis should be induced through the application of loop diuretics.

Patients with central insipidus diabetes can be treated with nasal or oral desmopressin while patients with nephrogenic insipidus diabetes can be treated with correction of potential precipitation factors and with a combination of thiazide diuretics and low sodium-low protein aimed at reducing the polyuria [68].

Potassium

Potassium is the main intracellular cation; 95-98% of the total body potassium is placed in the intracellular space, the remaining 2-5% is in the extracellular fluid compartment, including blood. Normal serum potassium level is between 3.5 and 5.0 mEq/L [69].

Maintaining this concentration is critical for many physiological processes (including cellular membrane potential, cellular volume, transmission of action potentials in nerve cells) [70] and several mechanisms play a role in potassium homeostasis, such as the intake, elimination, and balance between intracellular and extracellular fluid compartment.

Potassium daily intake is about 1 mEq/kg (60-100 mEq) [71]. Potassium's intestinal absorption is approximately 90% of the ingested. About 90% of its excretion is through kidney, which represents the most important factor for maintaining normal K+ balance. The remaining 10% is through gastrointestinal tract and sweat glands [72]. The active excretion of potassium, occurring in the distal tubule and the collecting duct, is controlled by aldosterone [73]. Its principal actions is changing epithelial sodium channel (EnaC) in the open configuration and increases its number in the cortical collecting duct (CCD). This implies that sodium reabsorption reassess, luminal electronegativity is increased and potassium secretion is enhanced [74].

Potassium distribution between intracellular and extracellular fluid compartments is attributed to Na+-K+-ATPase, a pump located in almost all cells, which brings 3 sodium ions out and 2 potassium ions inside the cell [75]. This concentration gradient across the membrane is mainly responsible for the resting potential of cellular plasma membrane. Many factors are involved in this working: serum pH, in particular alkalosis causes the potassium input into cells, acidosis causes the transition from intracellular to extracellular fluid compartments; insulin, b-adrenergic catecholamines, which both move K+ inside the cell [76].

Hypokalemia

Hypokalemia is defined as a serum potassium level of less than 3.5 mEq/L (3.5 mmol/L). Severe hypokalemia is a level of less than 2.5 mEq/L. Hypokalemia is a potentially life-threatening imbalance that may be iatrogenically induced.

Symptoms

Patients are often asymptomatic, especially in the case of mild hypokalemia [77]. Symptoms of hypokalemia are non-specific and predominantly related to muscular or cardiac function. Severe hypokalemia may cause:

- weakness
- fatigue,
- myalgia,
- muscle cramps
- constipation,
- psychological symptoms (e.g., psychosis, delirium, hallucinations, depression),
- rhabdomyolysis,
- bradycardia and acute respiratory failure due to muscle paralysis with cardiovascular collapse.

Cardiac arrhythmias are life-threatening complications that require immediate diagnosis and treatment. The ECG findings related to hypokalemia include inverted T waves, a U wave, ST depression and a wide PR interval [78-79].

Causes

Hypokalemia is common in cancer patients and its mechanisms include: inadequate potassium dietary, redistribution of potassium and potassium losses [80]. All these causes may contribute to hypokalemia in cancer patients (Table 7).

The reduced intake is often due to malnutrition. Again, the refeeding syndrome (RS) is associated to hypokalemia. RS is a common condition occurring in patients with severe malnutrition, which is characterized by electrolyte disorders, such as hypophosphatemia, acute vitamin B1 deficiency, volume overload, cardiac insufficiency, hyperglycemia and hypokalemia [81].

The redistribution of potassium between intracellular an extracellular fluid compartment depends on many factors: uptake of potassium by tumor cells, alkalosis, and drugs. For example, myelopoietic growth factors, often used in cancer patients, induce an acute hematopoietic cell production and a rapid uptake of potassium by the new cells [82]. A similar mechanism explains the hypokalemia due to a rapid cell proliferation in acute leukemia [83].

Potassium lost can be divided into renal and not-renal. The most common extra-renal losses are gastrointestinal losses due to drug-induced diarrhea and vomiting, infection, radiation enteritis, and visceral tumors: villous adenoma and neuroendocrine tumors [84]. Neuroendocrine tumors represent a heterogeneous group of neoplasms that in less than 10% occur with the carcinoid syndrome (CS). The clinical manifestations of CS and hypokalemia are due to serotonin and kallikrein hypersecretion that causes cutaneous flushing, secretory diarrhea, wheezing, tachycardia or hypotension heart failure, cramps and bronchial constriction [85]. A rare syndrome of watery diarrhea associated with hypokalemia and achlorhydria and it is due to hypersecretion of vasoactive intestinal polypeptide [86]. Renal losses of potassium in cancer patients is often related to Cushing syndrome. Cushing syndrome in 10-20% of cases are due to tumors producing ACTH, such as SCLC, medullary thyroid carcinoma, islet cell adenoma or carcinoma, pheochromocytoma, ganglioneuroma [87].

Normally cortisol is converted by 11β-hydroxysteroid dehydrogenase type 2 (11β-HSD2) to inactive cortisone for mineralocorticoid receptor (MR). In Cushing syndrome, the excess of cortisol induces a saturation of renal 11β-HSD2 and circulating cortisol can reach MR to induce hypokalemia [88]. Another rare case of hypokaliemia associated with hypertension is Conn syndrome [89].

Primary aldosteronism is characterized by polydipsia, polyuria, resistant hypertension, profound hypokalemia, due to the excessive and autonomous secretion of aldosterone by an aldosterone-producing adenomas or carcinoma [90].

However, increased potassium renal losses can be also caused by drug-related tubular toxicity. Many chemotherapy agents, in fact, induce renal injury: mitomycin-C, gemcitabine, platinum compounds, methotrexate, ifosfamide, antiangiogenic drug, bisphosphonates and interferon [91]. Ifosfamide can induce toxicity in any segment of the nephron, causing urinary loss of potassium and magnesium from distal tubule. Amphotericin B and Cisplatin may cause distal tubulopathy with urinary loss of potassium and magnesium [92]. Recently hypokalemia has also been described in patients treated with abiraterone acetate [93].

Renal function should be evaluated in all cancer patients (also in patients with normal serum creatinine levels) using the Cockcroft-Gault formula, in order to make drug dosage adjustments when necessary [94]. Furthermore, in order to prevent kidney damage, it is important to administer specific premedication and avoid co-administration of nephrotoxic drugs such as aminoglycosides, non-steroidal anti-inflammatory drugs, lithium, heparin anticoagulated or iodinated contrast media [95].

Thiazide diuretics and glucocorticoids can cause loss of potassium by the kidneys, too.

Patients, with multiple myeloma producing Bence Jones proteins, develop a progressive renal damage that leads to hypomagnesemia and hypokalemia. Acute non-lymphocytic leukemia often induces a renal tubular defect, perhaps due to lysozyme [96].

Table 7. Causes of hypokalemia

Gastrointestinals and Non-Renal Losses	• Poor food intake • Losses (diarrhea, vomiting, fistula, laxative abuse, villous adenoma) • Profuse sweating • Extended burns • Toxic epidermal necrolysis
Endocrine Disfunctions	• Excess of glucorticoids • Excess of mineralocorticoids
Renal Losses	• Metabolic alkalosis • Diabetic ketoacidosis • Use of diuretics • Osmotic diuresis • Renal tubular diseases (tubular acidosis, Liddle syndrome)
Redistribution of the Potassium Inside the Cell	• Drugs (catecholamines, nasal decongestants, insulin, beta2 agonists, theophylline, bicarbonate, verapamil) • Metabolic or respiratory alkalosis • Accidental or induced hypothermia • Barium intoxication
Causes Of Ipokalemia in the Oncological Patient	• REDUCED POTASSIUM ASSUMPTION -malnutrition, anorexia • excessive gastrointestinal loss -vomit (caused by chemotherapy) -diarrhea (caused by chemotherapy, cancer, surgery) • RENAL LOSSES -diuretici -ipercalcemia -ipomagnesemia - post-ostruttive diuresis -pharmaceuticals (amphotericin B, cisplatin, ifosfamide, glucocorticoids, monoclonal anti-EGFR antibodies, mTOR inhibitors, eribulin, abiraterone) • EXCESS OF MINERALCORTICOIDI - primary hyperaldosteronism (adenoma or adrenal carcinoma) - Renin-secreting tumors - ectopic secretion of ACTH • PSEUDOIPOKALIEMIA • USE OF GROWTH FACTORS AND VITAMIN B12

Hypokalemia should not be confused with pseudo-hypokalemia, which is typical of patients with marked leukocytosis (e.g., in acute myeloid leukemia) and can be avoided by storing the blood sample on ice or rapidly separating the serum from the cells [97].

Diagnosis

Diagnosis of hypokalemia is based on detection of low values of serum potassium and clinical conditions. The differential diagnosis is based on detection of increased serum potassium levels and patient's medical history to exclude the presence of pseudo-hypokalemia by evaluating the concomitant treatments and the presence of conditions that may cause potassium intracellular redistribution (taking insulin, diuretics, chemo-therapy, diarrhea, vomiting). Hypokalemia may also be secondary to metabolic alkalosis. Other laboratory values such as blood sugar, creatinine, magnesium levels, electrolytes in urine and acid-base balance should be evaluated (Figure 4) [98].

The renal potassium excretion in the 24-hour urine should be evaluated in order to establish whether hypokalemia is attributable to renal or extrarenal causes.

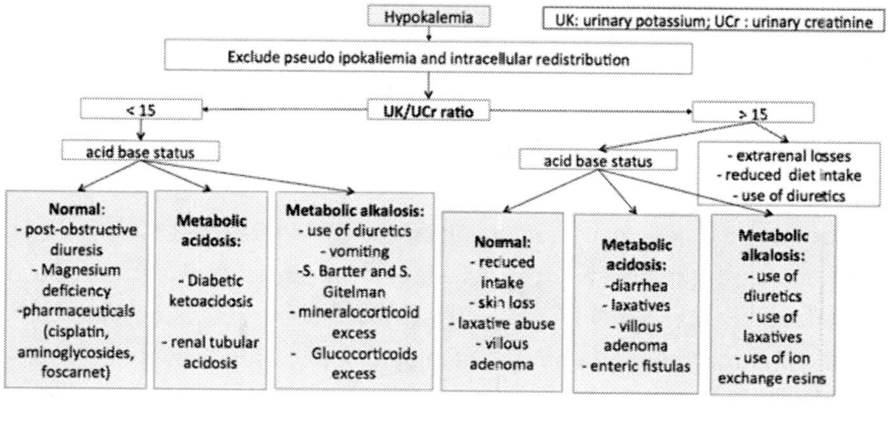

Figure 4. Hypokalemia diagnostic algorithm.

If the urinary potassium is >30 mEq/L, the cause is related to a urinary loss, potentially due to mineralocorticoid excess. If the urinary potassium is

<25 mEq/L, the cause is related to a loss of extra-renal potassium. The same information can be obtained by comparing the urinary potassium concentration with the urinary concentration of creatinine (Ucr). Values > 15 suggest the presence of renal causes of hypokalemia, while a ratio < 15 points towards extrarenal causes. In the latter case the evaluation of the acid-base state can help to differentiate the different pathological conditions [98].

Treatment

The management of hypokalemia should be based on symptoms and on serum potassium level. The aim of the treatment is preventing life-threatening complications, such as cardiac arrhythmias and respiratory failure and removing the cause.

Diagnosis and early treatment of concomitant hypomagnesemia is mandatory for effective treatment of hypokalemia, because it aggravates hypokalemia which becomes refractory to treatment with potassium [99].

Mild and moderate hypokalemia (serum potassium concentration, 3.0-35 mEq/L) is not a life-threatening condition and potassium oral route is preferred to intravenous for the lowest risk of rebound hyperkalemia. Recommended dose is 60-80 mEq/d of potassium chloride given orally in divided doses. However, it is necessary to re-check serum potassium level after replacement therapy and to adjust treatment accordingly. In patients with chronic hypokalemia, which do not respond to oral therapy, potassium-sparing diuretics, such as amiloride and spironolactone, can be consider [100].

Severe hypokalemia (serum potassium concentration <3.0 mEq/L), if asymptomatic, can also be treated with oral potassium (potassium chloride, 40 mEq, orally every 3-4 hours) [101]. Conversely when patients are unable to take oral medicine or a life-threatening complication occurs, intravenous potassium (10-20 mEq/h) should be administered [102]. A continuous cardiac monitoring should also be done in case of arrhythmias, digitalis toxicity, recent or ongoing cardiac ischemia. Administering 20 mEq/h of potassium chloride will increase serum potassium concentration by an average of 0.25 mEq/h, with associated mild hyperkalemia in only 2% of cases [103]. The highest concentration of KCl to be administered in a peripheral venous access is 40 mEq/L, because infusions of potassium are irritating and painful and can cause venous sclerosis. In patients with GFR <30 mL/min/1.73 m^2 (<0.5 mL/s/1.73 m^2), these rates should be decreased by 50%-80% with frequent (2- to 4-hour) reassessment of serum potassium concentration [104].

When hypokalemia is secondary to tumor activity, treating the cancer is necessary, in addition to symptomatic therapy for hypokalemia, in order to prevent the recurrence of symptoms.

The treatment of patients with CS is based on the somatostatin analogue. By inhibiting hormonal hypersecretion, somatostatin analogs reduce circulating hormone levels and ameliorate symptoms [105].

Primary aldosteronism due to a tumor, can be cured, when possible, with unilateral adrenalectomy, whereas patients can benefit from targeted pharmacotherapy with mineralocorticoid receptor antagonists, as spironolactone [106]. The treatment of choice for ectopic ACTH syndrome is complete resection of the tumors. There are many options to control severe hypercortisolemia (>30μg/dL): steroid-synthesis inhibitors (metyrapone, mitotane, trilostane, ketoconazole, aminoglutethimide) and glucocorticoid receptor antagonists (mifepristone) [107].

Grade 2 and 3 chemoradiotherapy-induced diarrhoea should be treated to prevent hypokaliemia. Probiotics, Loperamide and octreotide are most widely used drugs in these cases [108].

Hyperkalemia

Hyperkalemia is defined as a serum potassium level greater than 5.5 mEq/L. Potassium levels between 5.1 mEq/L to 6.0 mEq/L reflect mild hyperkalemia. Potassium levels of 6.1 mEq/L to 7.0 mEq/L represent moderate hyperkalemia while levels above 7 mEq/L reflect severe hyperkalemia and it might represent a life-threatening condition [109].

Symptoms

Patients are often asymptomatic for plasma potassium concentrations below 5.5 mEq/L.

The signs and symptoms of hyperkalemia include [109]:

- fasciculations
- cramps
- weakness
- ascending paralysis
- electrocardiographic alterations (pointed T waves, PR stretch elongation, enlarged QRS complex, reduced QT interval)
- arrhythmias (bradyarrhythmia, ventricular fibrillation, asystole) (Table 8).

Table 8. Approximate relationship between electrocardiographic changes due to hyperkalemia and plasma potassium levels

Plasma levels of potassium	Electrocardiographic alterations
Mild hyperkalaemia (5.5-6 mEq/l)	• Peaked T-waves, • Shortened QT interval • ST segment depression
Moderate hyperkalemia (6-7 mEq/l)	• Peaked T-waves • Prolonged PR segment • P waves disappearance
Severe hyperkaliemia (>7 mEq/l)	• enlarged and bizarre QRS complex with prolonged QRS interval • absence of waves P • intraventricular block • "sine wave" pattern sinusoidal pattern • ventricular fibrillation • asystole

Causes

In general, hyperkalemia occurs when there is an excessive intake, cells breakdown or abnormal elimination of potassium, secondary to aldosterone deficiency or to a renal parenchyma injury (Table 9).

Table 9. Causes of hyperkalemia

Pseudohyperkalemia	• incorrect sampling technique • *in vitro* hemolysis • laboratory error • leukocytosis • thrombocytosis
Increased Intake	
Increased Potassium Release from Cells	• massive tissue catabolism (hemolysis, diffuse trauma, rhabdomyolysis, chemotherapies) • drugs (beta-blockers, arginine, digital) • metabolic acidosis • insulin deficiency and hyperglycemia • severe muscular exercise • periodic paralysis (hyperkalemic variant) • cardiac surgery in hypothermia • pseudohyperkalemia
Reduction of Renal Excretion of Potassium	• kidney disease - acute or chronic renal failure - depletion of effective circulating volume - tubulopathies: hyperpotassiemic type I tubular acidosis - selective alteration of potassium excretion (acute transplant rejection, lupus nephritis, cyclosporine, analgesic nephropathy, lead poisoning) • corticosurrenal deficiency - iporeninemic hypoaldosteronism (diabetic nephropathy, chronic interstitial nephritis, drug nephropathy) - primitive hypohaldosteronism (M. of Addison) • use of potassium-sparing diuretics
Causes Of Iperkaliemia in the Oncological Patient	• effective circulating volume reduction • summary of luminous tissue • sepsis • surrenal insufficiency • chemotherapy drugs (cisplatin, ifosphamide, mitomycin c, gemcitabine, methotrexate, diphosphonate, interferon, octreotide).

Potassium intake alone is a very uncommon cause of hyperkalemia for an individual with normal kidney function, it could happen only with large infusions of KCl or extremely high oral doses (>160 mEq) of potassium [110].

Conversely, in patients with diabetes mellitus, renal insufficiency, or during treatment with medications that interfere with potassium excretion (e.g., potassium-sparing diuretics, angiotensin-converting enzyme [ACE] inhibitors and nonsteroidal anti-inflammatory drugs [NSAIDs]), or nutritional cancer therapy, rich on potassium, life-threatening hyperkalemia can occur [111].

Focus on Hyperkaliemia in Cancer Patients

Hyperkalemia in cancer patients may be due to several causes, some secondary to cancer or its treatment, other independent of the tumor (Table 8). An important cause of acute hyperkalemia in cancer patients is represented by the tumor lysis syndrome, an oncological emergency characterized by hyperuricemia, hyperkalemia, hyperphosphatemia, hypocalcemia, and azotemia, which appears 48–72 hours after the initial treatment (chemotherapy, radiotherapy, radiofrequency ablation) [112]. In high-grade hematologic malignancies it can also occur spontaneously [113]. It occurs most frequently in childhood cancers and hematological malignancies, while it is rare in adult solid tumors. [114-115]

Factors predisposing to tumor lysis syndrome are large tumor masses, neoplasms in rapidly growing, neoplasms sensitive to chemotherapy, preexisting renal failure and elevated lactate dehydrogenase (LDH), hyperuricemia and hyperazotemia [116]. The pathogenesis of the syndrome is related to stress effects of chemotherapy or radiotherapy on cellular metabolism [116]. The result is cell necrosis and the acute release of intracellular products into the systemic circulation. Elevated uric acid and calcium phosphate precipitate into the renal tubule and may cause inflammation, glomerular filtration rate reduction until acute renal injury, which aggravates these metabolic disorders and hyperkalemia. Furthermore, the increasing serum potassium can cause cardiac arrhythmias and lead to death; this risk can be exacerbated by low serum calcium and acidosis [117].

Hyperkalemia in cancer patients can be due to adrenal insufficiency due to metastasis in both adrenal glands. Although autopsy studies demonstrated adrenal glands metastasis in up to 40–60 percent of patients with disseminated lung or breast cancer clinical adrenal insufficiency is rarely reported, due to concomitant use of corticosteroids [118].

The few case-reports on Addisonian crisis due to metastatic adrenal infiltration were represented by patients affected by lung cancer or lymphoma [119-120].

Finally, in cancer patients with extreme leukocytosis or thrombocytosis can be seen pseudohyperkalemia, due to the escape of the potassium from platelets and leucocytes after a blood sample or the formation of a coagulum. In this setting, pseudohyperkalemia should be ruled out with the determination of plasma potassium instead of serum in a heparinized tube [121].

Diagnosis

Diagnosis of hyperkalemia is based on detection of increased serum potassium levels and on clinical conditions. Patients with hyperkalemia are often asymptomatic and the disorder is discovered as an incidental laboratory finding. Symptoms are related to lowering cell-resting action potential, inducing abnormal muscle, neurological and cardiac functions, until life-threatening cardiac dysrhythmias. Patients may report general fatigue and weakness, paresthesia, muscular paralysis and palpitations. Hyperkalemia can also appear only with electrocardiographic changes like peaked T-waves, decrease or absence of P waves, prolonged PR interval, bradycardia [122].

The differential diagnosis is based on history (potassium intake, medications), urine potassium, sodium and osmolality, trans tubular potassium gradient (TTKG), complete blood count, metabolic profile. If hyperkalemia is associated with an increase of creatinine and urea, creatinine clearance should be calculated because it may be due to renal failure. If it is associated with hyperuricemia, hyperkalemia, hyperphosphatemia, hypocalcemia, the cause may be a TLS. If TTKG > 10, it is usually secondary to excessive intake of potassium. A TTKG <10 is generally secondary to a mineralocorticoid deficiency. In this case, serum levels of renin and mineralocorticoid should be assayed [123].

Treatment

Treatment of hyperkalemia in cancer patients does not provide a specific therapy, and it depends on changes on the ECG, symptoms and degree of hyperkalemia.

The diagnosis of hyperkalemia requires:

- to assess the presence of a life-threatening condition requiring emergency treatment,
- to perform an ECG,
- to obtain a venous access, when necessary [124].

Patients with severe hyperkalemia and electrocardiographic changes due to hyperkalemia should be given immediate treatment.

Moderate hyperkaliemia can be treated with Potassium- binding resins, such as sodium polystyrene sulfate, which exchange sodium for potassium cations in the gastrointestinal tract [125].

Nevertheless, its slow onset of action, poor tolerability and potential toxicity for inducing colonic necrosis in the critically ill patients contraindicate its use for most patients. However, it remains a valuable drug for unstable or elderly patients, when dialysis is not possible [126].

For a correct management of hyperkalemia it is recommended [127-128]:

1. Eliminate all exogenous sources of potassium and, if possible, suspend drugs that may cause hyperkalemia.
2. Counteract cardiac effects of potassium: evaluate the symptoms and the ECG and in case of enlargement of the QRS administer calcium e.v. (e.g., 1fl calcium gluconate 10 ml) which can be repeated based on electrocardiographic changes.
3. To bring back potassium inside the cells: in asymptomatic patients a rapid correction of hyperkalemia can be obtained by administering [129-140]:

- 10% glucose solution 500 ml or 250 ml at 20% or 100 ml at 50% with 10 units of fast insulin and 5 cc of emagel to be infused in 30-60 minutes;
- Sodium bicarbonate (1 mEq / kg) in 10-20 minutes to be repeated after 5 min if the electrocardiographic abnormalities persist and the potassium values remain high. However, sodium bicarbonate should be used with caution in patients with heart failure or renal failure, where fluid retention may worsen.
- Beta-2 agonists: 10-20 mg salbutamol diluted in 4 ml of Physiological Sol and inhaled in 10 minutes. It should not be used in case of ischemic cardiomyopathy or arrhythmias.

These therapies can have a rapid effect, but only cause a temporary redistribution of potassium in the intracellular space.

Sodium bicarbonate and beta-2 agonists should not be used as monotherapy in the correction of hyperkalemia, but as adjuvant treatments [129].

4. Remove excess potassium (effects and reduction of plasma levels of potassium may be visible only after several hours) [131]:
    - Administer intestinal ion exchange resins (Kayexalate 15 g in 60 cc of water from 1 to 4 times/day per os or 50 g of resin in 50 ml of 20% sorbitol with 100-150 ml of water from the endorectal route). Resins should be used with caution in patients with heart failure and renal failure due to volume overload due to the high sodium content of these drugs.
    - Infuse liquids (200 ml/h) and diuretics (furosemide 40-80 mg). Use with caution in patients with heart failure due to fluid overload.
    - Dialysis in case of renal failure and if the resins and diuretics fail [132].

There is no evidence to support the use of diuretics in the acute treatment of hyperkalemia, therefore their use should be reserved only for the management of some chronic forms.

Plasma potassium concentrations should be frequently monitored during treatment (every 1-6 hours) in symptomatic patients with severe hyperkalemia; further monitoring of plasma potassium levels after therapeutic interventions and resolution of symptoms every 4 to 12 hours until normal plasma levels of potassium is recommended [133-134].

Magnesium

Magnesium is the second most prevalent intracellular cation. It is an essential cofactor for enzymes utilizing or synthesizing ATP, representing a fundamental cofactor necessary for the normal cells' functional, replication and energy metabolism processes and it is involved in muscular contractility and neuronal transmission and phosphate transfer [135].

About 99% of body magnesium is intracellular: 50–60% of the total body magnesium is in bone, 38% in soft tissues and only 1% is extracellular. Normal serum magnesium levels range between 1.5 and 1.9 mEq/L (1.7–2.2 mg/dl), more than 70% of plasma magnesium is in ionized form.

Magnesium is absorbed by the gastrointestinal tract. The adult human daily nutritional requirement is around 300-400 mg/day. Magnesium serum level is controlled mainly by kidney. Renal elimination of $Mg2+$ is passive through the glomerulus, reabsorption is passive in the ascending limb of the loop of Henle (60-70%), and active in the distal tubule and in the collecting duct (10%). It is influenced by many hormonal factors (PTH, calcitonin, glucagon, and vasopressin) and non-hormonal (acid-base changes, and potassium depletion) and plasma [$Mg2+$] that is the major regulator [136].

Hypomagnesemia

Hypomagnesemia is an electrolyte disturbance which occurs when magnesium serum level is less than 1.5 mEq/L and it is considered severe when serum level is <1 mg/dl. Hypomagnesemia is frequently found in hospitalized patients (7-12%), and is associated with an increased mortality [137].

Hypomagnesemia is often associated with other electrolyte abnormalities such as hypocalcaemia and hypokalemia, often refractory to other treatments. Low plasma levels of potassium associated with a condition of hypomagnesaemia are an important risk factor for the development of severe arrhythmias, therefore in critical patients magnesium is often corrected up to 2 mg/dl [138].

Symptoms

Symptoms usually do not occur until magnesium concentration falls below 1.2 mg/dl (0.49 mmol/L), although the severity of symptoms may not be correlated with serum magnesium levels [139].

Deficiency of magnesium causes weakness, muscle cramps, cardiac arrhythmia, increased irritability of the nervous system with tremors, athetosis, jerking, nystagmus and an extensor plantar reflex. In addition, there may be confusion, disorientation, hallucinations, depression, epileptic fits, hypertension, tachycardia and tetany (Table 10).

Table 10. Symptoms of hypomagnesemia

Cardiovascular	Electrocardiographic abnormalities Severe ventricular arrhythmia Hypersensitivity to the digital Hypertension
Neuromusculars	Muscle tremors Fascications Tetany Altered mental state (depression, psychosis) Ataxia Dizziness Convulsions
Electrolytic	Hypokalemia Hypocalcemia
Metabolic	Glucose intolerance/Hyperinsulinism Atherosclerosis
Bone	Osteoporosis

Electrocardiographic alterations may include lengthening of the PR and QT intervals, flattening or inversion of the T wave, loss of the upward concavity of the ST [140].

Causes

Hypomagnesemia can result from different causes. Insufficient magnesium intake, altered absorption, kidney magnesium losses are the main causes of hypomagnesemia in cancer patients (Table 11).

Prolonged nasogastric suction, diarrhea, malabsorption syndromes, extensive bowel resection, severe malnutrition are the main causes of altered absorption.

Many drugs can increase renal magnesium losses. Cisplatin administration with cumulative dosages exceeding 300 mg/m2 is associated with hypomagnesemia in up to 90% cancer patients. Cisplatin-induced hypomagnesemia mainly results from drug-induced distal renal tubular damage Hypomagnesemia due to cisplatin can persist years after therapy in cancer patients [141].

Thus, intravenous supplementation of magnesium on the day of cisplatin administration and 2–3 days after therapy is indicated as it would appear to be related to a decreased risk of cisplatin nephrotoxicity [142].

Some EGFR inhibitors may cause hypomagnesemia. In fact, EGFR activation is essential to Mg reabsorption in the kidney by the TRPM-6 channel [143].

A recent meta-analysis of 25 randomized clinical trials demonstrated that treatment with monoclonal anti-EGFR antibodies is associated with an incidence of hypomagnesemia of 34%; moreover, the use of Panitumumab would seem to be associated with a greater incidence than Cetuximab [144].

Furthermore, the finding of hypomagnesemia during treatment with Cetuximab in patients with metastatic colorectal carcinoma could represent a predictor of efficacy [145], although other studies have not confirmed these results.

Ifosfamide, aminoglycoside, and amphotericin B can also cause distal renal tubular damage, resulting in hypomagnesemia. Diabetes mellitus and hypercalcaemia of malignancy may also induce hypomagnesaemia [146].

Table 11. Causes of hypomagnesemia

Redistribution	• acidosis correction • re-feeding syndrome • catecholamines • • accelerated osteogenesis
Gastrointestinal Causes	• reduced income • malabsorption syndrome • protracted vomiting/diarrhea • • intestinal drainag /fistulae
Alcoholism	
Renal Losses and Renal Disorders	• reduced sodium reabsorption • infusion of saline diuretics • post-obstructive nephropathy • renal transplantation • dialysis • diuretic phase of acute renal failure • hereditary disorders (e.g., Bartter's syndrome, Gitelman's syndrome)
Causes Endocrine	• hyperparathyroidism • malignant hypercalcemia • hyperthyroidism • aldosteronism • SIADH • diabetes mellitus
Drugs	• diuretics • cytotoxic drugs (cisplatin) • EGFR inhibitors • antibiotics (aminoglycosides, anti-tuberculosis, immunosuppressants) • beta-adrenergic agonists • foscarnet • amphotericin B
Other	• Pancreatitis, burns, excessive sweating, pregnancy and lactation

Diagnosis

The earliest manifestations of hypomagnesemia are usually neuromuscular and neuropsychiatric disorders, often aspecific. Furthermore, symptomatic magnesium depletion is often associated with multiple biochemical abnormalities, including hypokalemia, hypocalcemia, and metabolic acidosis. As a result, hypomagnesemia is sometimes difficult to attribute solely to specific clinical manifestations [147].

The diagnosis is based on the history of gastrointestinal or renal losses or intake of some drugs. In cases of doubt between gastrointestinal and renal losses, the fractional excretion of magnesium (Fe-Mg), the measurement of the magnesium excretion in the 24-hour urine and the relationship between urinary calcium and creatinine (calcium-creatinine ratio) with a urine test should be determined (Figure 5).

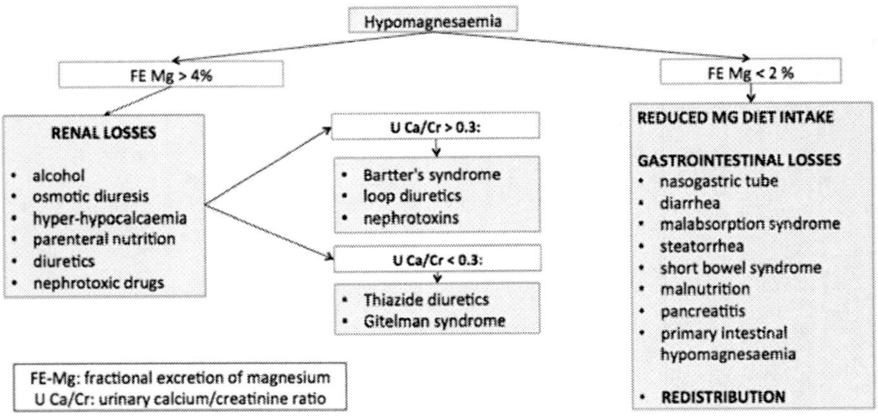

Figure 5. Diagnostic algorithm for hypomagnesaemia.

If urine magnesium concentration is greater than 2 mmol/day there is a renal wasting. In case of grade 3/4 hypomagnesemia, patients should receive appropriate and aggressive replacement therapy due to the high risk of cardiac arrhythmias and sudden mortality [148].

Treatment

In patients at risk of developing magnesium deficiency, laboratory indices and clinical symptoms should be assessed and any prophylactic treatment should be considered even in the presence of normal serum magnesium levels. The treatment of hypomagnesemia depends on the severity of clinical findings. Where possible the underlying diseases should be treated [149].

Oral administration of magnesium salts is preferred in asymptomatic patients (40 -60 mEq/day or 8-32 mEq/day in divided doses); however, diarrhea appears as a dose-limiting side effect. An initial dose of 12 mmol/day should be administered incrementally to 48 mmol/day.

Symptomatic patients should receive 1-4 g (8-32 mEq, up to a maximum of 1.0 mEq/kg) of magnesium e.v. sulfate, slowly infused in 12-24 hours (1 g/hour). This dose may be repeated if necessary to maintain magnesium levels at about 1.2 mg/dl.

To correct severe hypomagnesaemia, 4 to 6 g (32-48 mEq up to a maximum of 1.5 mEq/kg) of magnesium sulfate are often required.

The maximum infusion rate should be 8 mEq/h (1 g of magnesium sulfate per hour up to 100 mEq of magnesium (approximately 12 g of magnesium sulfate) in 12 hours in asymptomatic patients, up to 32 mEq of magnesium (4 g of magnesium sulfate) in 4-5 minutes in patients with symptomatic severe hypomagnesaemia [149].

Doses <6 g $MgSO_4$ can be administered in 8-12 h, while higher doses should be infused over a period >25 hours since the rapid intravenous administration of magnesium causes an increase in serum magnesium concentrations above physiological levels, increasing their renal excretion; therefore, given the slow distribution of magnesium in the tissues, the duration of the infusion is essential to obtain an adequate correction of hypomagnesemia. In case of intoxication, calcium e.v. (100-200 mg in 5-10 min) should be administrated to antagonize the neuromuscular and cardiovascular effects of magnesium [150].

Furthermore, in case of cisplatin-based chemotherapy, intravenous supplementation of magnesium on the day of cisplatin administration and 2–3 days after therapy is indicated.

Calcium, potassium and phosphate supplementation should be considered in patients with hypomagnesemia; there is also often a vitamin D deficiency that should be treated [149].

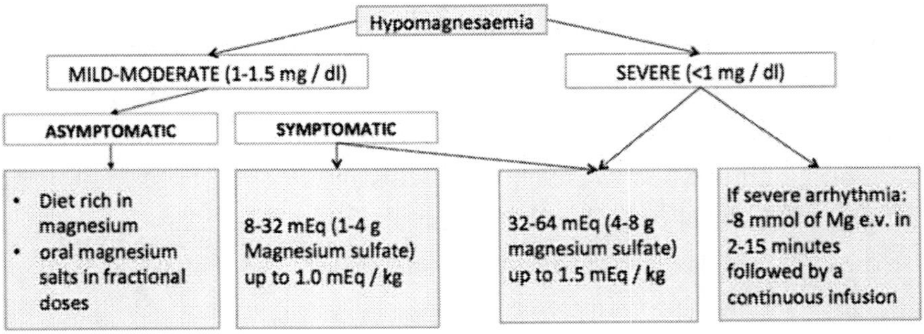

Figure 6. Therapeutic algorithm for hypomagnesaemia.

Hypermagnesemia

Hypermagnesemia is defined as a magnesium plasma concentration >2.2 mEq/L.

Causes

Hypermagnesemia is rare and usually iatrogenic (intravenous magnesium, magnesium-containing laxatives or anti-acids).

Diagnosis and Treatment

Clinical manifestations of hypomagnesaemia include hypotension, bradycardia, respiratory depression, depressed mental status, and ECG abnormalities as bradycardia, complete AV-block and, at the end, asystole [151]. Treatment should include discontinuation of magnesium intake in whatever form and hemodialysis may be necessary in severe cases. Symptomatic hypermagnesemia with cardiac arrhythmias, respiratory depression and hypotension calcium gluconate 10% is suggested. In severe cases hemodialysis may be necessary.

Phosphate

Phosphate is a crucial component of various cellular processes, being a component of the nucleic acids, DNA and RNA and being a fundamental part of adenosine triphosphate (ATP), that carry energy for most of cellular functions. Furthermore, it is an essential component of bone matrix. Phosphate is main intracellular anion, complexed or bound to proteins and lipids. Only 1% of total phosphate is extracellular fluid. Most of total body phosphate is localized in bone as part of the mineralized extracellular matrix providing mineral strength to bone and it represents the main accessible phosphate pool. Approximately 300 mg per a day of phosphate is mobilized from bone tissue. Excessive phosphate losses or insufficient intake leads to osteomalacia [152]. Normal serum phosphate concentration is a range between 3.0-4.5 mg/dl.

Phosphate homeostasis depends on several factors and its serum concentration is regulated by diet, hormones, calcium levels and pH. Most of the phosphorus derives from diet. Intestinal absorption of phosphorus can be modulated by the expression of transporters influenced by vitamin D and parathormone (PTH). However, the use of antacids, severe diarrhea or intestinal malabsorption can cause significant phosphate deficits.

Phosphorus excretion occurs mainly in kidneys and PTH, and Vit D modulate it [152].

High dietary phosphate intake and elevated PTH levels decrease renal phosphate absorption, thus enhancing renal excretion, while high vitamin D levels enhance renal phosphate absorption. PTH and vitamin D are the most important regulators of phosphate metabolism, the first favoring phosphate renal elimination, the second favoring phosphate intestinal absorption and bone deposit. Fibroblast growth factor 23 (FGF23) seems to have a role in phosphate metabolism, favoring phosphaturia. Overexpression of FGF23 associated with specific tumors seems to correlate with the syndrome of oncogenic osteomalacia, characterized by acquired hypophosphatemic rickets and renal phosphate wasting [153]. Furthermore, insulin favors intracellular shift of serum phosphate.

Hypophosphatemia

Hypophosphatemia is defined as a serum phosphate concentration <2.5 mg/dL (0.8 mmol/L). This electrolyte disturbance is most frequent in hospitalized patients, where hypophosphatemia is observed in 1-5% of patients and it is usually mild and asymptomatic. The incidence rises in individuals with alcoholism, diabetic ketoacidosis, or sepsis, with frequency rates of about 40-80% [154].

In advanced cancer patients seems to be a frequent electrolyte alteration and mild hypophosphatemia has been seems to correlate with poor outcomes. A recent study reported hypophosphatemia in about 70% of patients (50% of grade ≥2 and 20% grade 3) [155]. It can be related to tumor metabolism, clinical conditions and anticancer treatment. Furthermore, early post-operative hypophosphatemia seems to be a negative prognostic factor for cancer patients undergoing abdominal surgery, with higher risk of post-operative complications [156].

Symptoms

Clinical presentation of hypophosphatemia is often nonspecific. However, it can be different in patients, depending on cause, duration, and severity.

Mild hypophosphatemia (2-2.5 mg/dL), independently of onset speed (acute or chronic), is usually asymptomatic. Severe or chronic hypophosphatemia is more frequently symptomatic and presenting features are related to deficit of ATP and then energy generation or bone fragility such as weakness, bone pain, loss of bone density, fractures, rhabdomyolysis, until altered mental status, hemolysis, cardiac and respiratory failure in more serious cases [157]

Causes

Altered regulation of phosphate, is relatively common in cancer patients. It might depend on antineoplastic treatment of cancer conditions such as cachexia and malnutrition, causing calcium and vitamin D deficiency. The main pathogenic mechanisms that might cause hypophosphatemia are (Table 12):

- Inadequate intake
- Increased losses
- Cellular shift (from extracellular to intracellular space).

Table 12. Causes of hypophosphatemia

Inadequate Intake	• Magnesium deficiency • Vitamin D deficiency • Cachexia • Cushing's syndrome • Aluminium-containing antacids
Increased Losses	• Hyperparathyroidism • Renal tubular dysfunction (e.g., drugs, alcoholism, isolated proximal tubule phosphate wasting, Fanconi syndrome) • Chelation • Drugs (diuretics, glucocorticoids, aminoglycosides, antiretrovirals) • Hypercalcemia • Gastrointestinal losses (vomiting, diarrhoea)
Cellular Shift	• Diabetic ketoacidosis • Administration of glucose and insulin • Respiratory alkalosis • Refeeding after prolonged undernutrition • Catecholamine • Hungry bone syndrome • Diabetes
Causes Of Hypophosphatemia In The Oncological Patient	• Cachexia and malnutrition • Drugs (cisplatin, • Type of tumors (lymphoma, multiple myeloma, chondrosarcoma, osteoblastoma, hemangiopericytoma) • Tumor-induced osteomalacia (TIO)

Chemotherapy, in particular nephrotoxic agents such as cisplatin, might directly damage renal tubules causing phosphate wasting. Several target therapies (imatinib, sunitinib, dabrafenib) have been described to induce hyphosphatemia. However, the exactly incidence of hyphosphatemia in this setting and its clinical implications are still unknown [155-158]. Certain tumours might induce hypophosphatemia, mediated by different mechanisms. Multiple myeloma can directly damage renal tubules, resulting in phosphaturia and hypophosphatemia. Acute leukaemia might cause hypophosphataemia for inappropriate phosphaturia or because of the

'Warburg effect', due to an excessive consumption of glucose compared to healthy tissues to produce energy [159]. Processes such as glycolysis and the synthesis of ribose phosphates leads to a high consumption of phosphate resulting in hypophosphatemia. The syndrome of tumor-induced osteomalacia (TIO) is characterized by overproduction of FGF-23 resulting in phosphate wasting, hypophosphatemia, and osteomalacia. Most frequently, tumors causing TIO are chondrosarcoma osteoblastoma, hemangiopericytoma, ossifying fibromas, giant-cell tumors, and granulomas [160].

Diagnosis

Since symptoms of hypophosphatemia are often a specific, it is important for cancer patients monitoring this electrolyte's serum concentration in order to do no under evaluate and quickly correct it. Once assessed hypophosphatemia in cancer patients, a careful evaluation of concomitant medications, nutritional status, and medical history should be performed. Serum calcium, magnesium, albumin and kidney function should be also studied to reach a correct diagnosis of hypophosphatemia, in order to detect causes and begin the correct therapy (Figure 7).

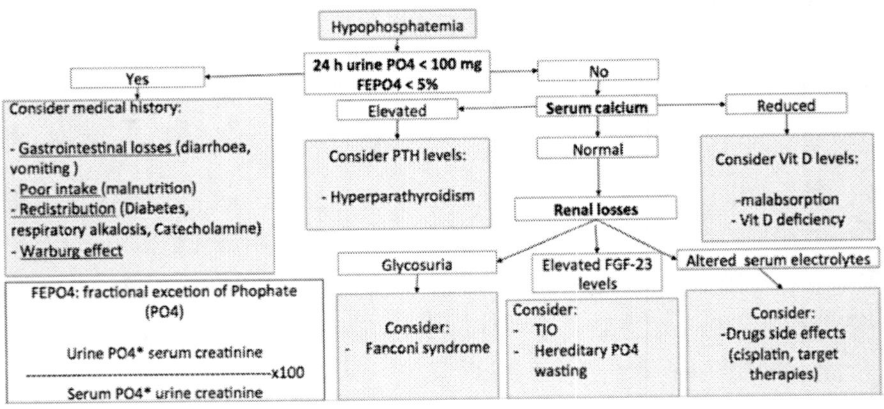

Figure 7. Diagnostic algorithm for hypophosphatemia.

Concomitant hypercalcemia, might suggest hyperparathyroidism and a chemistry panel including also PTH, and PTHrP should be performed.

In presence of patients with malabsorption, malnutrition, osteoporosis (for example in patients treated with hormonal therapies) especially if hypophosphatemia is associated with hypocalcemia, Vitamin D levels should be dosed. Normal serum calcium level might be correlated to increased renal losses and phosphate renal wasting (evaluating urine phosphorus concentration in 24-hour urine collection) should be considered. Measurement of serum FGF-23 levels might be performed in this case, in suspicion of TIO. However, this test is useful only in limited and selected cases.

When respiratory alkalosis is suspected, an arterial blood gas study should be performed [161].

Treatment

Treatment of hypophosphatemia depends on three aspects: cause, severity, and duration. Whether the cause of the hypophosphatemia is detected, it should be treated when possible. Treatment for hypophosphatemia is still controversial. When serum phosphate level is <2.0 mg/dL but >1.0 mg/dl, even in asymptomatic patients, oral phosphorus supplements is recommended. The aim is to maintain a phosphate level among 2 and 2.5 mg/dL, in order reduce and control symptoms [162]. When oral supplementation of phosphate is associated to vitamin D intake, the risk of hyperphosphaturia should be considered, since it might lead to calcium phosphate kidney stones production. In these cases, the association with thiazide diuretics should be consider in order to reduce urine calcium excretion. Intravenous phosphate supplements should be used only in patients with life-threatening hypophosphatemia (<1 mg/dL) or non-functional gastrointestinal syndromes, as it is associated with a high risk of hyperphosphaturia. In case of severe hypophosphatemia (< 1.0 mg/dL) or moderate hypophosphatemia (1.0–2.5 mg/dL) but symptomatic, patients should receive intravenous replacement therapy with an initial dose of 0.08-0.16 mmol/kg infused over 2-6 hours. After reaching phosphate serum levels above 1.0 mg/dl oral supplementation should be preferred [161].

Even if serum phosphate levels are low representative of total body phosphorus, it is necessary monitoring serum phosphate and calcium levels every 6 hours, to prevent overcorrection of hypophosphatemia and to maintain normal calcium concentration. The evaluation of urinary phosphorus excretion, might be consider as it seems to better indicate adequate phosphorous repletion. Treatment of concomitant electrolyte alteration should be obtained. Patients with vitamin D deficiency should receive vitamin D supplementation [162].

To improve the management of these patients a multidisciplinary evaluation i.e., recommended. Endocrinologists and surgeons should be involved in the management of patients with primary hyperparathyroidism. Gastroenterologists and nephrologists should be involved in case of gastrointestinal or renal losses, respectively.

Hyperphosphatemia

Hyperphosphatemia is defined as an elevated serum phosphate level greater than 4.5 mg/dl. It is considered significant when concentration is up to 5 mg/dL in adults and 7 mg/dL in children or adolescents. It is a rare electrolytic alteration in the general population; however, it is very frequent in patients with advanced chronic kidney disease, which incidence is at least 70% [163].

Symptoms

More commonly, patients with hyperphosphatemia have general symptoms or are asymptomatic. Often signs and symptoms such as muscle cramps, tetany, and perioral numbness or tingling, reported by patients with acute hyperphosphatemia result from concomitant hypocalcemia. In some cases, it might induce bone and joint pain, pruritus, rash and it might contribute to renal osteodystrophy.

In most cases, patients complain symptoms related to hyperphosphatemia. For example, patients with renal failure have uremic symptoms such as fatigue, shortness of breath, anorexia, nausea, vomiting, and sleep disturbances.

Hyperphosphatemia induce a progressive decreasing of vitamin D production, and it interferes in bone metabolism in particular with PTH-mediated bone resorption, causing hypocalcemia, that in rare cases can be life-threatening. Prolonged hyperphosphatemia favorites soft-tissue calcification, that can involve cardiac valves, eyes, joints, and vasculature and muscles [164]. In rare cases, hyperphosphatemia might result in calciphylaxis, a tissue ischemia due to calcification of small vessels with subsequent thrombosis.

Causes

The main cause of hyperphosphatemia in cancer patients is related to tumor lysis syndrome. However, it might occur for other reasons. Pathophysiology of hyperphosphatemia is based on three different pathogenic mechanisms:

- Increased or dysregulated phosphate intake (gastrointestinal absorption, exogenous administration),
- Reduction of phosphate renal excretion,
- Phosphate shift from intracellular to extracellular space (cellular release).

Excessive phosphate intake is a rare cause of hyperphosphatemia. In fact, homeostatic mechanisms are able to eliminate phosphate excess. However, in particular conditions such as impaired mechanisms of renal excretion, Vitamin D intoxication or an excessive intake of laxatives containing phosphate, an increased or dysregulated phosphate intake might hesitate in hyperphosphatemia. The main cause remains acute or chronic renal failure (especially when glomerular filtration rate lower than 25 ml/min), that induces decreased excretion of phosphate. Lymphoma thought enzyme 1-α hydroxylase's action might cause increased activity of vitamin D resulting in hypercalcemia and hyperphosphatemia.

Tumor lysis syndrome is the most frequent cause of hyperphosphatemia in cancer patients representing a potential fatal complication of antineoplastic therapy. It might compare in patients with high cell turn over neoplasms. It is characterized by a series of laboratory anomalies (hyperuricemia, hyperkalemia, hyperphosphatemia and hypocalcaemia) due the release of intracellular contents secondary to acute and massive cancer cell necrosis. It often occurs after antineoplastic therapies but sometimes it might happen spontaneously. The released intracellular metabolites (in particular nucleic acids, protein, and phosphorus, potassium) can hesitate in renal failure and serious cardiac arrhythmias up to multiple organ failure and death [164].

Table 13. Causes of hyperphosphatemia

Excessive Intake	• Intravenous or oral excessive supplementation • Vitamin D intoxication • Drugs (laxatives, • Milk-alkali syndrome
Reduced Excretion	• Renal failure • Hypoparathyroidism • Diphosphonate therapy • Acromegaly • Magnesium deficiency • Tumoral calcinosis • FGF23 deficiency
Cellular Shift	• Rhabdomyolysis • Haemolysis • Acidosis (metabolic or respiratory) • Malignant hyperthermia • Excessive bone resorption • Hypoinsulinemia
Causes of Hyperphosphatemia in the Oncological Patient	• Tumor lysis syndrome • Excessive intake • Type of tumors (lymphoma, Multiple myeloma)

Pseudo-hyperphosphatemia should be excluded in case of hemolyzed blood samples, hyperlipidemia, hyperbilirubinemia, and dysproteinemia due for example to multiple myeloma.

Diagnosis

Since symptoms of hyperphosphatemia are often aspecific or related to hypocalcemia, it is important for cancer patients monitoring this electrolyte's serum concentration, especially for patients with high cell turn over neoplasms to exclude presence of tumor lysis syndrome. A careful medical history is crucial to avoid the risk of vitamin D intoxication, laxative (Phospho-soda) abuse, rhabdomyolysis, and tumor lysis. Once assessed hypophosphatemia in cancer patients, it is crucial to assess serum calcium, magnesium, blood urea nitrogen (BUN), and creatinine concentrations (Figure 8). A low calcium concentration con be related to renal failure, hypoparathyroidism, and pseudohypoparathyroidism, while BUN and creatinine values are useful to detect renal failure. Concomitant elevated serum calcium level might be observed in case of vitamin D intoxication or milk-alkali syndrome. The dosage of PTH, thyroid stimulating hormone, creatinine kinase and vitamin D are useful for a correct differential diagnosis [165].

Treatment

Treatment approach of hyperphosphatemia should consider cause, severity, and duration.

Chronic hyperphosphatemia is often associated to renal failure. In these cases, treatment is based on limitation of oral phosphate intake. Dialysis should be considered in case of symptomatic irreversible and severe chronic or acute renal failure, especially when associated to hypocalcemia. When diet control is not effective at controlling hyperphosphatemia, the addition of phosphate binders, which mechanism of action is to inhibit gastrointestinal absorption of phosphate, should be considered. However, when calcium-containing binders are used, it should be necessary to monitor serum calcium and phosphate level. To favorite renal elimination of phosphates, loop diuretics may be employed, or saline and/or acetazolamide may be administered [166]. In rare cases of primary hypoparathyroidism, the treatment aim is to control hypocalcemia and usually the prescription of calcium and vitamin D are sufficient. In rare cases recombinant PTH injections can be considered [167]. When the cause of hyperphosphatemia is tumor lysis syndrome, the therapy should include correction of electrolyte disorders and uric acid lowering agents.

Tumor lysis syndrome should be prevented with abundant hydration, eventually loop diuretics and uric acid lowering agent (allopurinol or rasburicase) [168].

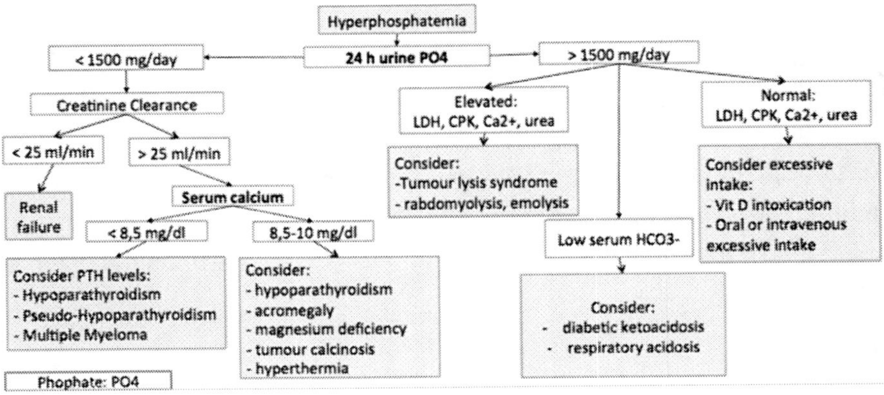

Figure 8. Diagnostic algorithm for hyperphosphatemia.

Calcium

Calcium is basically an extracellular ion and the plasma calcium levels range goes from 8.5 mg/dl to 10.5 mg/dl (2.1-2.5 mmol/L) [169]. Changes in acid–base status can alter calcium binding to proteins. In particular, an acute alkalosis increases binding and decreased ionized calcium and instead an acute acidosis has the opposite effect. These changes do not modify total calcium measurement.

Calcium is present in three forms: as a free ion (50%) or bound to plasma proteins and, in smaller quantities, in the form of diffusible complexes. The average nutritional intake of calcium is approximately 0.6-0.8 mg/day, 20–40% of the average intake of calcium of healthy adults is absorbed. The principal dietary source is dairy products [169].

Kidney excretes calcium and most of the calcium is reabsorbed by kidney (98% in the proximal tubules and a lesser amount by the ascending loop of Henle), with a loss of only about 2%. Loop diuretics and volume expansion decrease tubular resorption of calcium, whereas hypovolemia and thiazide diuretics have the opposite effect [170]. The amount of excreted calcium is directly proportional to urinary excretion of sodium and sulfate.

The most important regulation of calcium metabolism between bone and ECF involves the soluble portion of calcium in the bones. The bone remodeling process involves the breakdown of hydroxyapatite crystals by osteoclasts, a laying down of organic matrix by osteoblasts in the tunnels made by the osteoclasts and the mineralization of the organic matrix by hydroxyapatite crystals [171]. PTH has direct effects on bone (to increase osteoclastic- and osteocytic-mediated bone resorption that appears within minutes to hours, to promote the transfer of calcium across the osteoblast-osteocyte membrane without movement of phosphate; to influence the reabsorption increasing osteoclast activity, to stimulate the production of RANKL, a protein that plays a crucial role in osteoclast formation and functions and to inhibit osteoblastic role) and on kidney metabolism of calcium (enhanced renal tubule reabsorption of filtered Ca that occurs within minutes, decreasing renal phosphate reabsorption through the proximal tubules and involving in the activation of vitamin D) and indirect effects on gastrointestinal metabolism of calcium mediated by vitamin D [172].

Calcitonin also affects calcium metabolism acting as a counter balance to PTH determining hypocalcemia and hypophosphatemia. Calcitonin decreases the movement of calcium from the labile bone calcium pool (behind the osteoblast-osteocyte barrier) to the ECF. It, also, decreases bone resorption through an inhibitory effect on the osteoclasts. Calcitonin also increases renal excretion of calcium and phosphate [173]. The control of calcitonin secretion is mediated by calcium as well: increased calcium concentrations cause increased secretion of calcitonin.

A decrease in calcium concentration stimulates PTH secretion, which causes the synthesis of active vitamin D and increases intestinal absorption of calcium. A decline in phosphate concentrations results in decreased inhibition of the C-1 hydroxylation, which indirectly results in increased 1,25-vitamin D production and increased absorption of phosphate [174].

Vitamin D also affects the bone, promoting the movement of calcium ions from the labile pool into ECFs and the resorption of bone, as well as enhancing the effects of PTH on bone metabolism of calcium [175].

Calcium-mediated signaling pathways have also been shown to play crucial roles in carcinogenesis: transformation of normal cells to cancerous cells and progression of disease. In fact, the changes in calcium wave oscillation frequency can activate transcription factors such as nuclear factor of activated T cells resulting in modulation of cellular transcription [176].

Cancer cells can become dedifferentiated into cancer stem cells in the tumorigenic progress and calcium signaling is involved in the differentiation process either through the extracellular calcium-sensing receptor and/or alterations in intracellular calcium [177].

Furthermore, the intracellular calcium signaling plays an important role in cellular motility in particular during tumor invasion and metastasis, while the extracellular calcium signaling has been shown to be associated with bone metastasis. Moreover, calcium is involved in regulation of apoptosis and immune system especially with mechanism of cytosolic signals control [178].

Hypocalcaemia

Hypocalcaemia is defined as when serum ionized calcium is less than 8.5 mg/dl or less than 4.5 mmol/dl.

Symptoms

The severity of clinical signs and symptoms of hypocalcaemia correlates with the intensity and time of the onset and is influenced by acid–base status, hypomagnesaemia and sympathetic overactivity [179].

Clinical manifestations of hypocalcemia are due to alterations of the electrical potential of the cell membrane. Muscle cramps at the level of the back and leg disorders are frequent in these patients. Hypocalcaemia slow insidious onset may produce a mild diffuse encephalopathy and should be suspected in any patient with dementia, depression or psychosis not otherwise explicable.

Severe hypocalcemia with plasma calcium <7 mg/dL (<1.75 mmol/l) can cause tetany, laryngospasm or generalized convulsions. Latent tetany generally occurs with less severely reduced calcemia (7 to 8 mg/ dL; 1.75 to

2.20 mmol/l) and may be also present in 10% of healthy individuals [180].

Table 14. Symptoms of hypocalcemia

Acute	• Tetany • Paraesthesias (peri- orals and extremities) • Muscle contractions • Trousseau's sign • Chvostek's sign • Seizures • Laryngospasm • Bronchospasm • Prolongation of the QT section • Hypotension • Heart failure • Arrhythmias • - Papilledema
Chronic	• Ectopic calcifications (basal ganglia) • Extrapyramidal symptoms • Parkinsonism • Dementia • Subcapsular cataract • Dry skin

Arrhythmias or heart block may occasionally occur in patients with severe hypocalcemia.

The ECG typically shows a prolongation of the QTc interval and ST. It can also observe alterations of repolarization, such as a pointed shape of the T wave or its inversion [181].

Numerous other alterations are associated with chronic hypocalcemia, such as dry scaly skin, brittle nails, thickened hair, parkinsonism, cataract. In patients with idiopathic hypoparathyroidism candida infection is common (Table 14) [182].

Causes

Several factors might cause hypocalcemia in cancer patients [183] (Table 15).

A common cause of reduced plasma calcium (but not ionized calcium) is hypoalbuminemia.

Free fatty acid in the total parenteral nutrition, instead, can increase calcium and albumin binding [184], as well as alkalemia resulting in less ionized calcium without a change in total serum calcium. In this instance, despite of a normal serum calcium value, symptomatic hypocalcemia can occur due to the reduction of physiologically active calcium.

Potential causes of real hypocalcemia are renal failure determining the lack of hydroxylation of 25-hydroxycholecalciferol to calcitriol with a consequent reduction of gut absorption and renal tubular reabsorption of calcium [185].

The vitamin D deficiency [186], and reduction of PTH production are other important causes of hypocalcemia, especially for cancer patients. The PTH deficiency is more common after total thyroidectomy together with subtotal or total parathyroidectomy for malignancy. Risk factors for severe hypocalcemia after surgery include preoperative severe hypercalcemia, surgical removal of a voluminous adenoma or neck dissection and elevation of alkaline phosphatase [187].

A typical disorder post-parathyroidectomy is "hungry bone syndrome" that is observed in particular in metastatic parathyroid cancer but is common also in metastatic prostate cancer [188].

The syndrome in prostate cancer follows these events: osteoblastic metastases cause an increase of deposition of calcium and phosphate in bone and a decrease of serum concentrations of both ions. Then hypocalcemia determines stimulation of the parathyroid glands leading to secondary hyperparathyroidism with following hypophosphatemia [189].

Phosphate binds calcium and can reduce serum calcium concentration. In particular, retention of phosphate can be observed in patients with renal failure.

Moreover, several drugs (also chemotherapeutic agents) can be associated with hypocalcemia, often inhibiting the osteoclastic bone reabsorption including those used to treat hypercalcemia and those that altering the metabolism of vitamin D [190].

Table 15. Causes of hypocalcemia

Reduction of not ionized calcium	Hypoalbuminemia: nephrotic syndrome; liver disease; citrate in blood product
Reduction of ionized calcium	Total parenteral nutrition enriched of free fatty acid
Renal failure	nephrotoxic chemotherapy agent; post-renal obstruction; compression and infiltration by malignancy; tumor lysis syndrome; hyperuricemia; sepsis; contrast agent nephropathy
Vit D deficiency or resistance	inadequate dietary intake; reduced absorption due to hepatobiliary or intestinal malabsorption; liver disease;
PTH deficiency or resistance	subtotal or total parathyroidectomy; autoimmune disorders; abnormal parathyroid gland development; altered regulation of PTH
Concomitant electrolyte disorders	hypomagnesemia renal failure
Drugs	phenytoin; phenobarbital; rifampicin; calcium chelators; radiographic contrast agent; bisphosphonates; denosumab; cisplatin; 5-fluorouracil; leucovorin; nab-paclitaxel; estramustine; octreotide; imatinib; axitinib; panitumumab; cetuximab; furosemide; foscarnet; EDTA; cinacalcet
Extravascular deposition	hyperphosphatemia; osteoblastic metastases; pancreatitis

Zoledronic acid is a potent bisphosphonate, inhibiting osteoclast function, which delayed or prevented skeletal-related events in patients with bone metastases [191].

Denosumab is fully human anti-RANKL monoclonal antibody that decreases the incidence of skeletal-related events in metastatic bone disease [192].

In a report of 120 patients who received zoledronic acid for multiple myeloma or other malignant neoplasms, hypocalcemia was observed in 35% of patients [193]. Denosumab has a more potent bone resorption inhibitory activity than zoledronic acid, as shown by bone turnover markers [194].

The incidence of hypocalcemia and hypophosphatemia is higher in patients receiving such therapy compared to those receiving zoledronic acid, as demonstrated in the three registered studies [195].

In healthy individuals, severe hypocalcemia does not occur because of compensatory mechanisms: increased 1-alpha hydroxylation of vitamin D, increased secretion of PTH that leads to increased renal reabsorption of calcium and stimulation of osteoclastic bone resorption. Hanamura et al. identified co-administration with corticosteroids, pre-treatment hypocalcaemia (<2.37 mmol/L), and multiple bone metastases (>3) as risk factors for bisphosphonate-induced hypocalcaemia [196].

Calcium levels are often normal prior to initiating and administering subsequent doses of denosumab or bisphosphonates and should be monitored closely in the event of intercurrent gastrointestinal illness and renal impairment [197].

Chemotherapy and biological drugs may induce hypocalcemia. Among the others, cisplatin has an effect on renal tubular function, magnesium metabolism, bone resorption, and vitamin D potentially causing hypocalcemia [198].

In the classic case, hypocalcaemia is caused by excessive urinary loss and decreased renal up-take during high-dose cisplatin treatment. Proximal tubular damage leads to decreased reabsorption of cations. Chronic nephrotoxicity is characterized by a decrease of glomerular filtration rate and a slightly elevated but persistent magnesium, potassium and calcium excretion.

Cisplatin associated hypocalcaemia and hypercalciuria cannot be influenced by calcium supplementation [199].

Also, imatinib determines changes to renal and gastrointestinal handling of phosphate and calcium and it seems to target cells of the skeleton, stimulating the retention and sequestration of calcium to bone, leading to decrease circulating levels of these minerals [200].

Other drugs implicated in hypocalcaemia include axitinib, nab-paclitaxel (with an estimated hypocalcemia of about 33%), estramustine (estimated hypocalcemia of 20%), low doses of leucovorin/5-fluorouracil and octreotide (estimated hypocalcemia of 20%) [201]; cetuximab and panitumumab may increase the risk of hypocalcaemia [202].

Also, furosemide causes hypercalciuria and sometimes consequently hypocalcemia [203].

Calcium can also reduce for its extravascular deposition.

In fact, osteoblastic metastases use calcium during bone mineralization, activating a high calcium uptake, which can result in hypocalcaemia.

A retrospective analysis by Murray et al. found that prostate cancer patients with bone metastases have lower serum calcium, higher PTH and higher bone turnover markers than those with localized disease. The correlation between hypocalcaemia and hyperparathyroidism is strongest in patients with bone metastases and progressive disease. These findings indicate that osteoblastic metastases, in particular metabolically active disease, can cause hypocalcaemia. Cancer treatment often involves exposure to corticosteroids and cytotoxics which are toxic to cells including osteoblasts and osteocytes [204].

Also, hyperphosphatemia due to hypoparathyroidism can be responsible to hypocalcemia also due to deposition of calcium, as calcifications, in the kidney, brain, eye or vasculature. Bone turnover is decreased, and bone mass is increased [205].

Moreover, a chronic pancreatitis, can result in pancreas stones and consequently reduction of serum calcium; an acute pancreatitis instead causes hypocalcemia through sequestration of calcium by saponification with fatty acids [206].

Finally, magnesium-deficient patients show a defective parathyroid hormone (PTH) secretion that lead to hypocalcemia [207].

Diagnosis

Serum calcium is partially linked to proteins so it is recommended to always correct serum calcium levels as a function of albuminemia:

CORRECTED CALCIUM (mg/dL): serum calcium (mg/dL) + 0.8 * (4-patient's albumin)

CORRECTED CALCIUM (mmol/L): serum calcium (mmol/L) + 0.02 * (40-albumin measured g/L)

Alternatively, ionized calcium can be measured.

Hypocalcemia is often asymptomatic. The symptoms are primarily determined by ionized fraction but generally do not appear unless the serum ionized calcium concentration drops below 2.8 mg/dl (0.7 mmol/l), which usually corresponds to a serum total calcium concentration of 1.8–1.875 mmol/l (7.0–7.5 mg/dl) [208].

In addition of calcium, serum albumin and total protein as well as phosphate, vitamin D, plasma PTH and renal function should be measured.

Measurement of 24-hour or fractional excretion of calcium may also be useful. Further investigation of parathyroid, renal, liver or gastrointestinal failure should proceed as appropriate (Figure 9 and Table 16)

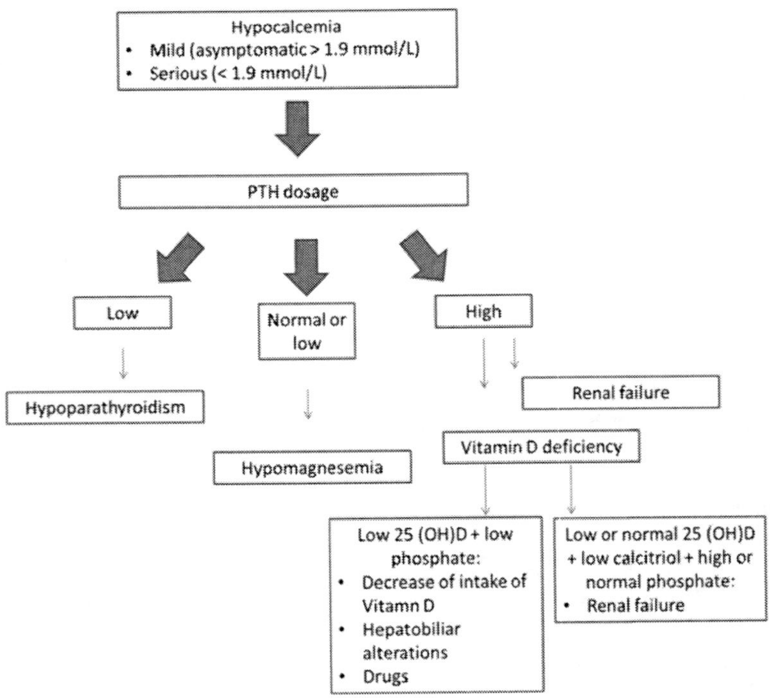

Figure 9. Diagnostic approach to the patient with hypocalcemia.

Table 16. Lab variations depending on hypocalcemia etiology

	PTH	Corrected Calcium	Phosphate	Mg	25(OH)D	1,25 (OH) 2D	Creatinine
Hypoparathyroidism	Low	Low	High	Normal	Normal	Normal or low	Normal
Hypomagnesemia	Normal or low	Low	Normal	Low	Normal	Normal	Normal
Vitamin D deficiency	High	Low or normal	Low or normal	Normal	Low	Normal or low	Normal
Chronic renal disease	High	Low	High	High or Normal	Normal or low	Low	High

Treatment

Acute, symptomatic hypocalcaemia should be treated with intravenous calcium slow pushes generally over 5-10 minutes (10 ml formulations of 10% calcium gluconate diluted in 50-100 ml of 5% dextrose) (90 mg calcium per 10 mL).

To avoid extravasation, calcium gluconate should be administered via a central venous catheter [209]. In addition, simultaneous oral calcium and calcitriol supplementation should be administered (0.25 to 1 mcg/day). Type of vitamin D formulation used depends on the diagnosis. Who has poor sunlight exposure or dietary insufficiency would benefit from cholecalciferol, those with renal failure should be given calcitriol [210].

Furthermore, any concomitant serum abnormalities, such as hypomagnesemia or alkalosis should be corrected [211].

During parenteral calcium gluconate infusion, cardiac function should be monitored, particularly in patients receiving digoxin, because of the risk of cardiac arrhythmias related to a rapid correction of hypocalcemia [212].

Signs and symptoms should guide the infusion rate, and ionized calcium levels should be measured every 1-2 hours.

Severe acute hypocalcemic tetany is treated initially with calcium gluconate intravenous infusion (10 ml of 10% solution in 10 minutes-bolus) followed by infusion of 1 to 3 mg of calcium gluconate in 500 ml of D5W-isotonic solution plus oral supplements of calcium (3 mg) and 2 to 3 g of dehydrocholecalciferol plus 1-2 mg of magnesium, if hypomagnesemia is present. In the following 12-24 hours repeated infusions or alternatively the addition of a continuous infusion, may be required.

Conversely, the treatment of hypoparathyroidism consists of the symptoms control, maintaining the calcium levels within a range between 2.00 and 2.12 mmol/L and the achievement of a calcium - phosphate ratio below 4.4 mmol/L without the development of hypercalciuria and precipitation of calcium salts in soft tissues [212].

Usually a vitamin D analogue is used such as calcitriol at a dose of 0.5 mcg/day with an increase in dose every 4 to 7 days until medium- to low calcemia levels are reached [213].

Thiazide diuretics decrease urinary calcium excretion due to increased distal tubular reabsorption: the administration of these drugs together with a low phosphate diet (avoiding dairy products, meat, cola drinks, eggs, and canned foods) can be considered [214].

Measurement of serum calcium, phosphorus concentration and creatinine should be performed weekly during initial administration and then every four months after stabilization of the dose [215].

Recent studies have demonstrated the efficacy of supplemental calcium and/or vitamin D, in minimizing the occurrence of hypocalcemia and subsequent emergency room visits and hospital readmission.

The oral calcium and vitamin D supplements can take a role in the prevention of postoperative hypocalcemia and in increasing the likelihood of a safe and early discharge from the hospital as demonstrated by Docimo et al. [216].

In chronic hypocalcemia oral supplements of calcium and vitamin D are recommended, in addition to the correction of hypomagnesemia [217].

Calcium carbonate and calcium citrate (at the dosage of 1 or 2 g of essential calcium three times a day) are considered the drugs of choice, containing the highest ratio of essential calcium (40 and 28% respectively) and being readily absorbed.

Furthermore, calcium and calcitriol supplementation usually normalizes asymptomatic electrocardiographic changes.

Finally, if hypocalcaemia is due to the malabsorption of vitamin D, the underlying cause should be treated (for example the incentive of a gluten-free diet in the celiac patient) [218]. Magnesium correction corrects hypocalcaemia related to low levels of magnesium [219].

Daily calcium (500 mg/day) and vitamin D (1000 UI/day) supplementation is also recommended during treatment with zoledronic acid in cancer patients, nevertheless hypocalcemia can still occur. Moreover, since patients with pre-existing hypocalcemia are susceptible to the development of severe symptomatic hypocalcemia, any pre-existing electrolyte imbalances should be treated before starting a bisphosphonate and regular electrolyte monitoring is recommended [220].

Vitamin D insufficiency requires correction with ergocalciferol (vitamin D2) or cholecalciferol (vitamin D3). The ergocalciferol can be administered at a dose of 50,000 IU a week or twice a week with a three-month reassessment of vitamin D levels, until normal levels of 25 (OH) D.

Alternatively, 300,000 IU of ergocalciferol can be administered intramuscularly, with the first two doses after three months and the following every six months [211].

Cholecalciferol is more potent than ergocalciferol; administration of 100,000 IU of vitamin D3 every 3 months is effective in maintaining an adequate level of 25 (OH) D.

Hypercalcaemia

Hypercalcaemia is defined as a serum calcium higher than 10.5 mg/dl. Hypercalcaemia is commonly associated with advanced cancer and poor prognosis [221].

Symptoms

Many patients with mild hypercalcemia are asymptomatic and the condition is often discovered incidentally during routine laboratory investigations [221].

It has widespread systemic effects including malaise, lethargy, constipation and abdominal pain and/or renal symptoms and signs: polyuria, polydipsia, nycturia, thirst, kidney stones and rarely renal failure and nephrocalcinosis. Moreover, hypercalciuria with nephrolithiasis is common.

Neurological complications are observed especially when calcium is >12 mg/dl (>3.00 mmol/l) and they are characterized by skeletal muscles weakness, emotional lability, confusion, delirium, psychosis, stupor and coma.

Asymptomatic hypercalcemia represents the most frequent clinical presentation of primary hyperparathyroidism. Nephrolithiasis is also common, in particular when the hypercalciuria is long-lasting.

Conversely, severe or long-lasting secondary hyperparathyroidism sometimes causes bone pain, in particular in patients on dialysis. Bone pain derives by the increased osteoclastic activity by PTH hyperstimulation with thinning of the bone, fibrous degeneration, the formation of cysts and nodules of fibrosis.

Causes

Hypercalcemia depends on several causes in cancer patients (Table 17).

To define hypercalcemia it is necessary to exclude several factors that can alter the ratio of bound to free calcium. Marked hyperglobulinemia will increase measured total calcium without altering ionized levels and therefore will not produce symptoms of hypercalcemia.

Acidemia decreases the affinity of albumin for calcium, thus increasing ionized, calcium without changing total calcium levels [222].

Primary hyperparathyroidism is probably the most common cause of hypercalcemia in the general population. It is a generalized disorder characterized by inappropriately high PTH and high serum calcium. Hyperparathyroidism-induced hypercalcemic crisis (HHC) is sometimes due to a single parathyroid carcinoma (PC) [223].

HCC, although rare, is typically associated with 10% of PC cases. The patients are often symptomatic due to elevated levels of PTH. In particular PTH levels are 3- to 10-times higher than normal value and serum calcium-levels is above the upper normal limit [224].

Table 17. Causes of hypercalcemia

Increase of total and not ionized calcium	Hyperglobulinemia
Increase of ionized and not total calcium	Acidemia
Increase of total and ionized calcium	- *Primary hyperparathyroidism*: parathyroid adenoma (MEN1 and 2a); parathyroid carcinoma; Familial hypocalciuric hypercalcemia; Isolated familial hyperparathyroidism - *Secondary hyperparathyroidism:* chronic hypocalcemia, especially due to renal failure; lithium - *Drugs:* lithium; thiazide diuretics; calcium containing antacids; vitamin A; estrogens; growth hormone; Vitamin D intoxication; theophylline - *Malignancy:* tumor production of PTHrP; osteolytic metastatic disease; ectopic activity of calcitriol; the excessive production of PTH - *Immobilization:* spinal cord injury; neurological diseases; pathological fracture; orthopedic surgery - *Miscellanea:* chronic granulomatous disorders; hyperthyroidism; acromegaly; pheochromocytoma; adrenal insufficiency; parenteral nutrition

Secondary hyperparathyroidism, instead, is due to low levels of activated vitamin D or intestinal malabsorption syndrome that stimulate the parathyroid to secrete PTH [225].

Furthermore, also hypercalcemia can be caused by drugs, sometimes indirectly through an increase of PTH. In particular lithium appears to increase the secretion of PTH, but can also unmask mild primary hyperparathyroidism [226].

Another important cause of hypercalcemia is malignancy, especially in hospitalized patients. Cancer-related hypercalcemia is one of the most common life-threatening metabolic disorders. It occurs in 20% to 30% of patients with cancer during the course of the disease and can be related to different mechanism, which depends on tumour type, too [227].

Some factors produced by the tumor are responsible to osteoclastic activation and bone destruction. In particular, they include parathormone-related peptide (PTHrP) that: acts on osteoblasts, increasing synthesis of

RANKL, with subsequent activation of osteoclasts and calcium release into the bloodstream; determines an increase of renal calcium reabsorption. PTH secretion results in pseudo-hyperparathyroidism, and it has no impact on the parathyroid glands, which remain normal or are even reduced in size [228].

Moreover, PTHrP, that leads the same receptors of PTH, does not seem to have a major influence on the production of the active form of Vitamin D [229].

Squamous cells head and neck carcinomas, renal cell, ovarian, endometrial, breast cancer, hepatocarcinoma, cholangiocarcinoma, colo-rectal cancer, neuroendocrine tumors, GIST and HTLV-1-associated lymphomas are frequently characterized by hypercalcemia (systemic hypercalcemia) [230-231-232-233].

Furthermore, osteolytic metastases are often associated with calcium release from bone determining hypercalcemia. This mechanism is considered the second more common cause of hypercalcemia, counting for approximately 20% of malignancy-related hypercalcemia. Metastatic bone lesions stimulate PTHrP through the release of local factors such as transforming growth factor β (osteolytic hypercalcemia) [234].

Considering multiple myeloma, lymphotoxin, interleukin-1 (IL-1), interleukin-6 (IL-6), hepatocyte growth factor (HGF), macrophage inflammatory protein (MIP-1alfa) and receptor activator of nuclear factor kappa B ligand (RANKL) facilitate bone remodeling and resultant hypercalcemia (Table 18 and Table 19) [235].

Table 18. Neoplasms most frequently associated with the onset of hypercalcemia

Neoplasms most frequently associated with hypercalcemia	
Multiple myeloma	40-50%
Breast cancer	>20%
Squamous pulmonary neoplasia	20%
Renal cell carcinoma	20%
Transitional cell urothelial carcinoma	5%
Gynecological neoplasms	5%
Head and neck tumors and esophageal carcinoma	5%

Table 19. Malignancy-related hypercalcemia

Osteolytic metastases	Breast carcinoma Multiple myeloma Lymphoma Leukemia
Systemic hypercalcemia (PTHrP)	Squamous cell carcinoma Renal cell carcinoma Bladder cancer Breast cancer Ovarian cancer Non-Hodgkin's lymphoma CML Leukemia Lymphoma
1,25-dihydroxyvitamin D	Lymphoma (Non-Hodgkin, Hodgkin) Ovarian dysgerminoma
PTH ectopic secretion	Ovarian cancer Lung cancer Papillary thyroid cancer

The third cause includes ectopic activity of 1-alpha-hydroxylase and the formation of calcitriol, that promotes intestinal calcium absorption and bone resorption. This mechanism is common in lymphomas (lymphoma-associated calcitriol production) and in some ovarian germ cell tumors.

Ectopic hyperparathyroidism, which is characterized by PTH production by non-parathyroid tumors, represents the fourth mechanism and it has been described in ovarian, lung, thyroid, neuroendocrine tumors, hepatocarcinoma, cholangiocarcinoma, leukemias and thymomas [236] or in rare cases PTH can be secreted by parathyroid carcinoma [237].

This paraneoplastic hypercalcemia can develop metastatic calcification involving multiple organs, especially lungs, potentially resulting in pulmonary edema [238].

Furthermore, the immobilization, in particular prolonged bed rest, which is common in advanced cancer patient, can cause hypercalcemia resulting in the acceleration of bone resorption. Hypercalcemia develops within days or weeks after starting bed rest in patients with spinal cord injury, neurological diseases, pathological fracture or patients underwent orthopedic surgery [239].

Diagnosis

Hypercalcaemia, acting via the calcium-sensing receptor, impairs the concentrating ability of the renal tubule to produce polyuria and volume depletion. The latter reduces the glomerular filtration rate and increases proximal tubular reabsorption of sodium, which carries calcium with it [240].

Hypercalcemia can be classified as mild, moderate and severe (Table 20).

Table 20. Classification of hypercalcemia

Mild	Moderate	Severe
<12mg/dL	12-14mg/dL	>14 mg/dL
<3 mmol/l	3- 3,5 mmol/l	>3,5 mmol/l
Often asymptomatic. Not required acute correction	It may be well tolerated, but may become symptomatic if the increase in calcemia is rapid requiring timely intervention	Always symptomatic; required urgent intervention due to the high risk of arrhythmias and coma

In some cases, it is useful to carry out the following selected laboratory tests:

- Concentration of BUN and creatinine (in order to monitor renal function)
- Immunoreactive parathyroid hormone (iPTH): iPTH is increased in parathyroid diseases while it is typically low or unmeasurable in malignant hypercalcemia
- the hormone related to parathyroid (rPTH) if available
- 1,25 di-hydroxy-vitamin D in patients with haematological malignancies
- serum concentration of phosphate and magnesium.

Electrocardiographic monitoring it's also important for the possible appearance of alterations such as:

- absent or shortened ST segment, shortened QT, widened QRS complex but lengthened T wave duration, prolonged PR interval, bundle branch block, Brugada syndrome (in predisposed individuals), and brady/dys-arrhythmias leading to cardiac arrest when serum calcium exceeds 15 mg/dl.

Significant hypercalcemia can cause specific electrocardiogram changes mimicking an acute myocardial infarction [241] (Table 21).

In general, primary hyperparathyroidism is usually characterized by hypercalcemia, hypophosphatemia and excessive bone resorption.

Serum calcium is rarely above 12 mg/dl, but the ionized free calcium is almost always high. In patients with hyperparathyroidism, PTH is inappropriately high (i.e., in the absence of hypocalcemia).

In presence of renal insufficiency, it may be difficult to distinguish primary from secondary hyperparathyroidism. In summary an elevated or high-normal PTH value is indicative of primary hyperparathyroidism. A low or low-normal value of PTH is indicative of non-parathyroid hypercalcemia. When hyperparathyroidism leads to an increase in bone turnover, the serum alkaline phosphatase is frequently increased [242].

Table 21. Lab exams associated with specific causes of malignant hypercalcemia

	PTH	**PTHrP**	**1,25 (OH)2D**	**25(OH)D**	**Phosphorus**
PTH-related	High	High	High	Low or normal	Low
1,25(OH)2D-related	Low	Low	High	Low or normal	Low
PTHrP-related	Low	High	Low or normal	Any value	Low
Vitamin D intoxication	Low	Low	High	High	Normal or high

In case of secondary hyperparathyroidism, radiographic examination usually shows the presence of bone cysts, a salt and pepper appearance of the skull and a subperiosteal bone resorption at the distal phalanges and clavicle.

Hypercalcemia may be associated with hypophospahtemia, hypophophaturia, metabolic alkalosis, hypochloremia, hypoalbuminemia, PTH level undetectable or greatly reduced and high levels of cAMP and urinary excretion of cAMP.

However, the diagnosis can be based on the individuation of PTH-rP. A serum calcium >12 mg/dl usually indicates the presence of a tumor or some other causes of hypercalcemia outside hyperparathyroidism.

Treatment

Treatment should be directed to the underlying cause and depends on the presence of symptoms, and on the severity of hypercalcemia. When the symptoms are mild and calcium in plasma is below 11.5 mg/dl (<2.88 mmol/l), it is often acceptable to correct only the underlying disorder whenever possible.

When the serum calcium level exceeds 15 mg/dl (3.75 mmol/l) or in presence of severe clinical signs of hypercalcemia, a direct treatment in order to reduce plasma levels of calcium is required [243].

Restoring adequate intravascular volume is fundamental to improve glomerular filtration rate and decrease passive sodium and calcium reabsorption from the proximal tubule [244].

Normal saline infusion: adequate hydration reduces serum calcium levels by an average of 0.25 mmol per liter. Re-hydration with 2-3 L of isotonic saline solution/day is recommended together with monitoring of electrolyte levels [245].

The majority of patients diagnosed with hypercalcaemia are dehydrated due to calcium-induced polyuria and fluid deprivation for nausea: hydration should begin with 100/120 ml/h intravenous or subcutaneously (adjusted for a urine output of 100–150 mL/h) [246].

Caution should be exercised when administering isotonic solution to patients with congestive heart failure or anuria, as fluid overload may occur. However, fluids alone determine normocalcemia in only 30% of patients.

Loop diuretics: the use of furosemide may be considered although overall efficacy is limited and may increase dehydration and the volume depletion and electrolyte abnormalities (monitor potassium, phosphorus and magnesium). Therefore, the treatment with furosemide could be considered for patients with heart failure and in whom it is necessary to increase diuresis [247].

Mobilization and diet: mobilization slows the loss of bone calcium due to immobility. A low calcium diet for the control of hypercalcemia with high levels of 1,25 (OH) D3 is not recommended because it may worsen the patient's malnutrition status. Patients should be allowed to freely drink water [248].

It has been suggested that the administration of salmon calcitonin (from 4 to 8 IU/kg s.c or i.m. every 12 hours; doses can be increased up to 6 to 8 international units/kg every six hours) can control the severe hypercalcaemia associated with malignancy even in patients with renal disease in which the primary treatment with intravenous saline is not advisable. In fact, calcitonin inhibits osteoclast activity and determines an increase in renal calcium excretion [249].

The drop in serum calcium (estimated maximal drop in calcium of 2 mg/dl) commonly happens within 4 h after administration.

Usually the duration of administration does not exceed 48 hours in order to reduce the risk of tachyphylaxis and the reaction; however infusion frequency are individualized to the hypocalcemic response [250].

Calcitonin administration lowers the calcium more quickly also than bisphosphonates and it could be used in presence of bisphosphonate resistance. It often produces normocalcemia within 12 to 24 hours, but it rapidly loses efficacy [251].

Calcitonin can be also used initially with bisphosphonates in cases of severe symptoms and very high calcium levels to incur a rapid response and allow time for the bisphosphonates to work. The usual dose of calcitonin is 100 units subcutaneously 3 times a day for 1 to 2 days [252].

If calcitonin loses its efficacy, it may be suspended for 2 days and then it is possible the re-administration [253].

The addition of 20-40 mg of prednisone p.o. daily or 200–400 mg daily of hydrocortisone every 6 hours for 3–5 days effectively controls hypercalcemia in the majority of patients with haematological malignancy, vitamin D intoxication, idiopathic hypercalcemia of infancy and sarcoidosis. Glucocorticoids decrease extra-renal calcitriol production in lymphoma or myeloma, increase renal excretion, and inhibit osteoclastic resorption from bone. Some patients with myeloma, lymphoma, leukemia or advanced breast cancer respond to 40-60 mg/day of prednisone. However, since the response to glucocorticoids requires several days and more than 50% of patients with hypercalcemia due to malignancies seem to not respond to glucocorticoids, an alternative treatment is usually approached [254].

Bisphosphonates (clodronate, etidronate (first generation), pamidronate, zoledronic acid, ibandronate (second generation)) represent an effective therapy for hypercalcemia through increased bone resorption. They inhibit bone turnover, directly, by inhibiting the recruitment and activity of osteoclasts, and indirectly, by stimulating osteoblasts to secrete an inhibitor of osteoclast formation. [255]

Bisphosphonates are now widely used as first-line therapy in combination with saline and furosemide for the treatment of hypercalcemia associated with malignancy.

Currently the first-generation or nonnitrogen-containing bisphosphonates are less commonly administered [256].

In the literature, the efficacy of pamidronate in restoring normocalcemia ranges between 40% and 70%, depending on the dose used (60-90 mg) and baseline serum calcium concentration; with a median duration of 4 weeks. It seems to be safe in patients with renal failure and can decrease plasma concentration of calcium in 5-7 days.

Early trials demonstrated pamidronate (60 mg over 24 hours) to be more effective in correcting hypercalcemia of malignancy than etidronate (70 percent versus 41 percent) or clodronate [258].

It is possible to start with 60 mg i.v. if the serum calcium concentration is up to 13.5 mg/dL (3 to 3.4 mmol/L) and 90 mg (maximal calcium response) for higher levels. Serum calcium concentrations begin to decrease in one or two days. Doses should not be repeated before seven days [259].

Zoledronic acid has a safety profile similar to pamidronate [260] and it is significantly more effective in reducing serum calcium (range 87-88%) with a duration of response longer than pamidronate (32-43 vs 18 days respectively). ZOL is administered at a dose of 4 mg over at least 15 minutes.

Bisphosphonate determine a reduction of serum calcium in approximately 12 hours, with a nadir in 4 to 7 days. Calcium levels can be checked 1 week after bisphosphonate infusion. In case of incomplete response, the infusion can be repeated. The use of bisphosphonates will result in a normocalcemic state for most patients. Without anticancer treatment, however, the hypercalcemia will likely recur within 2 to 4 weeks and the bisphosphonate treatment will need to be repeated. Recently, ibandronate, at the doses of 4 or 6 mg, has been introduced especially in patients with breast or hematological cancer. A randomized trial comparing ibandronate and pamidronate showed a comparable activity of the two drugs in reducing calcium levels (77 and 76% of response for ibandronate and pamidronate, respectively), while the median duration of response appeared to be longer for ibandronate (14 versus 4 days) [262].

Denosumab, a human monoclonal antibody, is an agent able to interfere with RANKL-RANK pathways [263], thus working through decreasing osteoclast activity and bone resorption [264].

Increasing evidence showed the utility of denosumab for the management of hypercalcemia of malignancy, particularly in patients with persistent hypercalcemia despite bisphosphonates [265].

Furthermore denosumab, unlike bisphosphonates, is not secerned by kidney, and so there is no restriction in patients with chronic kidney disease. However, in this setting of patients, the effect of denosumab may be higher, and it would be chosen a lower dose (half) [266].

Then an omission or suspension of administration if clearance of creatinine is <30 ml/min is recommended. The standard dose of denosumab is 120 mg subcutaneously that could be repeated no earlier than 1-week from the previous administration [267].

Conclusion

Electrolyte disorders are common in cancer patients and may contribute to worsen prognosis, since they interfere with anticancer treatment management. In fact, the development of electrolyte abnormalities may be associated with symptoms that can negatively affect the quality of life and may prevent chemotherapeutic regimens. Thus, the prompt diagnosis and treatment of these disorders are crucial for the care of cancer patients.

References

[1] Berardi R, Rinaldi S, Caramanti M, Grohè C, Santoni M, Morgese F, Torniai M, Savini A, Fiordoliva I, Cascinu S. 2016. "Hyponatremia in cancer patients: Time for a new approach." *Crit Rev Oncol Hematol* 102:15-25.

[2] Ingles Garces AH, Ang JE, Ameratunga M, Chénard-Poirier M, Dolling D, Diamantis N, Seeramreddi S, Sundar R, de Bono J, Lopez J, Banerji U. 2018. "A study of 1088 consecutive cases of electrolyte abnormalities in oncology phase I trials." *Eur J Cancer* 104:32-38.

[3] Masilamani S, Kim GH, Mitchell C, Wade JB, Knepper NA. 1999. "Aldosterone-mediated regulation of ENaC alpha, beta, and gamma subunit proteins in rat kidney." *Journal of Clinical Investigation* 104: R19–R23.

[4] Schneider EG, Radke KJ, Ulderich DA, Taylor Jr. RE. 1985. "Effect of osmolality on aldosterone secretion." *Endocrinology* 116: 1621–1626.

[5] Hall JE, Granger JP, Smith Jr. MJ, Premen AJ. 1984. "Role of renal hemodynamics and arterial pressure in aldosterone 'escape'." *Hypertension* 6: 1183–1192.

[6] Robertson GL. 1995. Posterior pituitary. In Felig P, et al. (eds) *Endocrinology and Metabolism*. New York: McGraw-Hill pp 385–432.

[7] Knepper MA. 1997. "Molecular physiology of urinary concentrating mechanism: regulation of aquaporin water channels by vasopressin." *American Journal of Physiology* 272: F3–F12.

[8] Acher R. 2002. "Water homeostasis in the living: molecular organization, osmoregulatory reflexes and evolution." *Annales d'endocrinologie* (Paris) 63: 197–218.

[9] Toney GM, Chen QH, Cato MJ, Stocker SD. 2003. "Central osmotic regulation of sympathetic nerve activity." *Acta Physiologica Scandinavica* 177: 43–55

[10] Beltowski J and Wojcicka G. 2002. "Regulation of renal tubular sodium transport by cardiac natriuretic peptides: two decades of research." *Med Sci Monit* 8:RA39-52.

[11] Cappuccio FP, Strazzullo P, Giorgione N, Iacone R, Farinaro E, Buckley MG, Miller MA, Sagnella GA, Macgregor GA, Mancini M. 1991. "Renal tubular sodium handling and plasma atrial natriuretic peptide, renin activity and aldosterone in untreated men under normal living conditions." *European Journal of Clinical Investigation* 21: 40–46.

[12] Ghali JK. 2008. "Mechanisms, risks, and new treatment options for hyponatremia." *Cardiology* 111:147-57.

[13] Palmer BF. 2003. "Hyponatremia in patients with central nervous system disease: SIADH versus CSW." *Trends Endocrinol Metab* 14:182–187.

[14] Castillo JJ, Vincent M, Justice E. 2012. "Diagnosis and management of hyponatremia in cancer patients." *Oncologist* 17: 756-65.

[15] Berghmans T, Paesmans M, Body JJ. 2000. "A prospective study on hyponatraemia in medical cancer patients: epidemiology, aetiology and differential diagnosis." *Support Care Cancer* 8: 192-7.

[16] Sengupta A, Banerjee SN, Biswas N M, Jash D, Saha K, Maji A, Bandyopadhyaya A, Agarwal S. 2013. "The Incidence of Hyponatraemia and Its Effect on the ECOG Performance Status among Lung Cancer Patients." *Journal of clinical and diagnostic research* 7:1678-82.

[17] Rawson NS and Peto J. 1990. "An overview of prognostic factors in small cell lung cancer. A report from the Subcommittee for the Management of Lung Cancer of the United Kingdom Coordinating Committee on Cancer Research." *Br J Cancer* 61: 597-604.

[18] Berardi R, Caramanti M, Fiordoliva I, Morgese F, Savini A, Rinaldi S, Torniai M, Tiberi M, Ferrini C, Castagnani M, Rovinelli F, Onofri A, Cascinu S. 2015. "Hyponatraemia is a predictor of clinical outcome for malignant pleural mesothelioma." *Support Care Cancer* 23:621-6.

[19] Schutz FA, Xie W, Donskov F, Sircar M, McDermott DF, Rini BI, Agarwal N, Pal SK, Srinivas S, Kollmannsberger C, North SA, Wood LA, Vaishampayan U, Tan MH, Mackenzie MJ, Lee JL, Rha SY, Yuasa T, Heng DY, Choueiri TK. 2014. "The impact of low serum sodium on treatment outcome of targeted therapy in metastatic renal cell carcinoma: results from the International Metastatic Renal Cell Cancer Database Consortium." *Eur Urol* 65:723-30.

[20] Kim HS, Yi SY, Jun HJ, Lee J, Park JO, Park YS, Jang J, Kim HJ, Ko Y, Lim HY, Kang WK. 2007. "Clinical outcome of gastric cancer patients with bone marrow metastases." *Oncology* 73:192-7.

[21] Choi JS, Bae EH, Ma SK, Kweon SS, Kim SW. 2015. "Prognostic impact of hyponatraemia in patients with colorectal cancer." *Colorectal Dis* 17:409-16.

[22] Dhaliwal HS, Rohatiner AZ, Gregory W, Richards MA, Johnson PW, Whelan JS, Gallagher CJ, Matthews J, Ganesan TS, Barnett MJ. 1993. "Combination chemotherapy for intermediate and high grade non-Hodgkin's lymphoma." *Br J Cancer* 68:767-74.

[23] Jeppesen AN, Jensen HK, Donskov F, Marcussen N, von der Maase H. 2010. "Hyponatremia as a prognostic and predictive factor in metastatic renal cell carcinoma." *Br J Cancer* 102:867-72.

[24] Berardi R, Caramanti M, Castagnani M, Guglielmi S, Marcucci F, Savini A, Morgese F, Rinaldi S, Ferrini C, Tiberi M, Torniai M, Rovinelli F, Fiordoliva I, Onofri A, Cascinu S. 2015. "Hyponatremia is a predictor of hospital length and cost of stay and outcome in cancer patients." *Support Care Cancer* 23:3095-101.

[25] Berardi R, Santoni M, Newsom-Davis T, Caramanti M, Rinaldi S, Tiberi M, Morgese F, Torniai M, Pistelli M, Onofri A, Bower M, Cascinu S. 2017. "Hyponatremia normalization as an independent prognostic factor in patients with advanced non-small cell lung cancer treated with first-line therapy." *Oncotarget* 8:23871-23879.

[26] Rondon-Berrios H and Berl T. 2016. "Vasopressin receptor antagonists: characteristics and clinical role". *Best Pract Res Clin Endocrinol Metab* 30:289–303.

[27] Verbalis JG, Goldsmith SR, Greenberg A, Korzelius C, Schrier RW, Sterns RH, Thompson CJ. 2013. "Diagnosis, evaluation, and treatment of hyponatremia: expert panel recommendations." *Am J Med* 126:S1-42.

[28] Pasovski G, Vanholder R, Allolio B, Annane D, Ball S, Bichet D, Decaux G, Fenske W, Hoorn EJ, Ichai C, Joannidis M, Soupart A, Zietse R, Haller M, van der Veer S, Van Biesen W, Nagler E. 2014. *Hyponatraemia Guideline Development Group.*

[29] Clinical practice guideline on diagnosis and treatment of hyponatraemia." *Nephrol Dial Transplant* 29 Suppl 2:i1-i39.

[30] Grohé C, Berardi R, Burst V. 2015. "Hyponatraemia--SIADH in lung cancer diagnostic and treatment algorithms." *Crit Rev Oncol Hematol* 96:1-8.

[31] Feldman BJ, Rosenthal SM, Vargas GA, Fenwick RG, Huang EA, Matsuda-Abedini M, Lustig RH, Mathias RS, Portale AA, Miller WL, Gitelman SE. 2005. "Nephrogenic syndrome of inappropriate antidiuresis". *N Engl J Med* 352:1884-90.

[32] Sorensen JB, Andersen MK, Hansen HH. 1995. "Syndrome of inappropriate secretion of antidiuretic hormone (SIADH) in malignant disease." *J Intern Med* 238:97–110.

[33] Otsuka F, Hayashi Y, Ogura T, Hayakawa N, Ikeda S, Makino H, Ota Z. 1996. "Syndrome of inappropriate secretion of antidiuretic hormone following intrathoracic cisplatin." *Intern Med* 35: 290–4.

[34] Berardi R, Santoni M, Rinaldi S, Nunzi E, Smerilli A, Caramanti M, Morgese F, Torniai M, Savini A, Fiordoliva I, Onofri A, Pistelli M, Taccaliti A, Cascinu S. 2016. "Risk of Hyponatraemia in Cancer

Patients Treated with Targeted Therapies: A Systematic Review and Meta-Analysis of Clinical Trials." *PLoS One* 11:e0152079.

[35] Fried LF and Palevsky PM. 1997. "Hyponatremia and hypernatremia." *Med Clin North Am* 81:585–609.

[36] Oren RM. 2005. "Hyponatremia in congestive heart failure." *Am J Cardiol* 95: 2B–7B.

[37] Papadakis MA, Fraser CL, Arieff AI. 1990. "Hyponatraemia in patients with cirrhosis." *Q J Med* 76: 675–88.

[38] Kurtz I and Nguyen MK. 2005. "Evolving concepts in the quantitative analysis of the determinants of the plasma water sodium concentration and the pathophysiology and treatment of the dysnatremias." *Kidney Int* 68:1982-1993.

[39] Gillum DM and Linas SL. 1984. "Water intoxication in a psychotic patient with normal renal water excretion." *Am J Med* 77: 773–4.

[40] Stuart CA, Neelon FA, Lebovitz HE. 1980. "Disordered control of thirst in hypothalamic-pituitary sarcoidosis." *N Engl J Med* 303:1078–82.

[41] Palevsky PM, Rendulic D, Diven WF. 1993. "Maltose-induced hyponatremia." *Ann Intern Med* 118: 526–8.

[42] Hillier TA, Abbott RD, Berrett EJ. 1999. "Hyponatremia: evaluating the correction factor for hyperglycemia." *Am J Med* 106: 399– 403.

[43] Goh KP. 2004. "Management of hyponatremia." *Am Fam Phys* 69:2387–2394.

[44] Petereit C, Zaba O, Teber I Grohé C. 2011. "Is hyponatraemia a prognostic marker of survival for lung cancer?." *Pneumologie* 65:565-71.

[45] Bartter FC and Schwartz WB. 1967. "The syndrome of inappropriate secretion of antidiuretic hormone." *Am J Med* 42: 790–806.

[46] Schrier RW. 2006. "Body water homeostasis: clinical disorders of urinary dilution and concentration." *J Am Soc Nephrol* 17:1820–1832.

[47] Peri A, Grohé C, Berardi R, Runkle I. 2017. "SIADH: differential diagnosis and clinical management." *Endocrine* 55:311-319.

[48] Verbalis JG. 2006. "AVP receptor antagonists as aquaretics: Review and assessment of clinical data." *Cleve Clin J Med* 73:S24 –S33.

[49] Petereit C, Zaba O, Teber I, Luders H, Grohe C. 2013. "A rapid and efficient way to manage hyponatremia in patients with SIADH and small cell lung cancer: treatment with tolvaptan." *BMC Pulm Med* 13:55 30.

[50] Peri A. 2013. "Clinical review: the use of vaptans in clinical endocrinology." *J Clin Endocrinol Metab* 98:1321-32.

[51] Cuesta M, Garrahy A, Thompson CJ. 2016. "SIAD: practical recommendations for diagnosis and management." *J Endocrinol Invest* 39:991–100.

[52] Palevsky PM, Bhagrath R, Greenberg A. 1996. "Hypernatremia in hospitalized patients." *Ann Intern Med* 124:197-203.

[53] Kraft MD, Btaiche IF, Sacks GS, Kudsk KA. 2005. "Treatment of electrolyte disorders in adult patients in the intensive care unit." *Am J Health Syst Pharm* 62:1663-82.

[54] Adroguè HJ and Madias EN. 2000. "Hypernatremia." *N Eng J Med* 342: 1493–1499.

[55] Snyder NA, Feigal DW, Arieff AI. 1987. "Hypernatremia in elderly patients. A heterogenous, morbid, and iatrogenic entity." *Ann Intern Med* 107: 309–19.

[56] Kahn T. 2000. "Hypernatremia in Hospitalized Patients: A Sequel of Inadvertent Fluid Administration—Reply." *Arch Intern Med* 160:1537-1538.

[57] Robertson GL. 1984. "Abnormalities of thirst regulation." *Kidney Int* 25: 460–9.

[58] Lindner G, Kneidinger N, Holzinger U, Druml W, Schwarz C. 2009. "Tonicity balance in patients with hypernatremia acquired in the intensive care unit." *Am J Kidney Dis* 54:674-9.

[59] Gipstein RM and Boyle JD. "Hypernatremia complicating prolonged mannitol diuresis." *N Engl J Med* 272:1116-7.

[60] Loh JA, Verbalis JG. 2007. "Diabetes insipidus as a complication after pituitary surgery." *Nat Clin Pract Endocrinol Metab* 3:489-94.

[61] Negro A, Regolisti G, Perazzoli F, Davili S, Sani C, Rossi E. 1998. "Ifosfamide-induced renal Franconi syndrome with associated

nephrogenic diabetes insipidus in an adult patient." *Nephrol Dial Transplant* 13:1547–9.

[62] Delaney V, de Pertuz Y, Nixon D, Bourke E. 1987. "Indomethacin in streptozocin-induced nephrogenic diabetes insipidus." *Am J Kidney* Dis 9:79–83.

[63] Bockenhauer D and Bichet DG. 2017. "Nephrogenic diabetes insipidus." *Curr Opin Pediatr* 29:199.

[64] Garofeanu CG, Weir M, Rosas-Arellano MP, Henson G, Garg AX, Clark WF. 2005. "Causes of reversible nephrogenic diabetes insipidus: a systematic review." *Am J Kidney Dis* 45: 626–37.

[65] Strange K. 1992. "Regulation of solute and water balance and cell volume in the central nervous system." *Journal of the American Society of Nephrology* 3: 12–27.

[66] Liamis G, Filippatos TD, Elisaf MS. 2016. "Evaluation and treatment of hypernatremia: a practical guide for physicians." *Postgrad Med* 128:299-306.

[67] Rose BD. *Clinical physiology of acid-base and electrolyte disorders.* 5th ed. New York, NY: Mcgraw-Hill; 2001.

[68] Palevsky PM. 1998. Hypernatraemia. In Greenberg A (ed.) *Primer on Kidney Diseases.* San Diego: Academic Press pp 64–71.

[69] Lien YH, Shapiro JI, Chan L. 1990. "Effects of hypernatremia on organic brain osmoles." *J Clin Invest* 85:1427-35.

[70] Sands JM, Bichet DG, American College of P, American Physiological S. 2006. "Nephrogenic diabetes insipidus." *Ann Intern Med* 144:186-94.

[71] Kratz A, Ferraro M, Sluss PM, Lewandrowski KB. 2004. "Case records of the Massachusetts General Hospital. Weekly clinico-pathological exercises. Laboratory reference values." *N Engl J Med* 351:1548-63.

[72] Pfennig CL, Slovis CM. 2012. "Sodium disorders in the emergency department: a review of hyponatremia and hypernatremia." *Emerg Med Pract* 14:1-26.

[73] Curtis CJ, Niederman SA, Kansagra SM. 2013. "Availability of Potassium on the Nutrition Facts Panel of US Packaged Food." *JAMA Intern Med* 173:828-829.

[74] Sica DA, Gehr TW, Yancy C. 2003. "Hyperkalemia, congestive heart failure, and aldosterone receptor antagonism." *Congest Heart Fail* 9:224–9.

[75] Giovacchini G, Nicolas G, Freidank H, Mindt TL, Forrer F. 2011. "Effect of amino acid infusion on potassium serum levels in neuroendocrine tumour patients treated with targeted radiopeptide therapy." *Eur J Nucl Med Mol Imaging* 38:1675-82.

[76] Eleftheriadis T, Leivaditis K, Antoniadi G, Liakopoulos V. 2012. "Differential diagnosis of hyperkalemia: an update to a complex problem." *Hippokratia* 16:294-302.

[77] Gennari FJ. 2002. "Disorders of potassium homeostasis. Hypokalemia and hyperkalemia." *Crit Care Clin* 18:273–288.

[78] Clausen T and Everts ME. 1989. "Regulation of the Na,K-pump in skeletal muscle." *Kidney International* 35:1–13.

[79] Krishna, GG; Miller, E; Kapoor, S. 1989. "Increased blood pressure during potassium depletion in normotensive men." *The New England Journal of Medicine* 320:1177–82.

[80] Lim S. 2007. "Approach to hypokalemia." *Acta Med Indones* 39:56-64.

[81] Kishimoto C, Tamaru K, Kuwahara H.Tall. 2014."P waves associated with severe hypokalemia and combined electrolyte depletion." *J Electrocardiol* 47:93-4.

[82] Yushui Ma, Likun Hou, Fei Yu, Gaixia Lu, Shanshan Qin, Ruting Xie, Huiqiong Yang, Tingmiao Wu, Pei Luo, Li Chai, Zhongwei Lv, Xiaodong Peng, Chunyan Wu, Da Fu. 2017. "Incidence and physiological mechanism of carboplatin-induced electrolyte abnormality among patients with non-small cell lung cancer." *Oncotarget* 8:18417–18423.

[83] Grasso S, Ferro Y, Migliaccio V, Mazza E, Rotundo S, Pujia A, Montalcini T. 2013. "Hypokalemia during the early phase of refeeding in patients with cancer." *Clinics* (Sao Paulo) 68:1413-5.

[84] Viens P, Thyss A, Garnier G, Ayela P, Lagrange M, Schneider M. 1989. "GM-CSF treatment and hypokalemia." *Ann Intern Med* 111:263.

[85] Adams PC, Woodhouse KW, Adela M, Parnham A. 1981. "Exaggerated hypokalaemia in acute myeloid leukaemia." *Br Med J (Clin Res Ed)* 282:1034–5.

[86] Stolinsky DC. 1978. "Emergencies in oncology. Current management." *West J Med* 129:169-76.

[87] Bendlow J, Apps E, Jones LE, Poston GJ. 2008. "Carcinoid syndrome." *European J of Surg Oncol* 34:289-296.

[88] Ikuta S, Yasui C, Kawanaka M, Aihara T, Yoshie H, Yanagi H, Mitsunobu M, Sugihara A, Yamanaka N. 2007. "Watery diarrhea, hypokalemia and achlorhydria syndrome due to an adrenal pheochromocytoma." *World J Gastroenterol* 13:4649-52)

[89] Thomas T, Zender S, Terkamp C, Jaeckel E, Manns MP. 2013. "Hypercortisolaemia due to ectopic adrenocorticotropic hormone secretion by a nasal paraganglioma: a case report and review of the literature." *BMC Res Notes* 6:331.

[90] Torpy DJ, Mullen N, Ilias I, Nieman LK. 2002. "Association of hypertension and hypokalemia with Cushing's syndrome caused by ectopic ACTH secretion: a series of 58 cases." *Ann N Y Acad Sci* 970: 134-144.

[91] Venkateswaran R, Hamide A, Dorairajan LN, Basu D. 2013. "Reninoma: a rare cause of curable hypertension." *BMJ Case Rep* pii: bcr2012008367.

[92] Born-Frontsberg E, Reincke M, Rump LC, Hahner S, Diederich S, Lorenz R, Allolio B, Seufert J, Schirpenbach C, Beuschlein F, Bidlingmaier M, Endres S, Quinkler M; Participants of the German Conn's Registry. 2009. "Cardiovascular and cerebrovascular comorbidities of hypokalemic and normokalemic primary aldosteronism: results of the German Conn's Registry." *J Clin Endocrinol Metab* 94:1125-30.

[93] Lameire NH, Flombaum CD, Moreau D, Ronco C. 2005. "Acute renal failure in cancer patients." *Ann Med* 37:13–25.

[94] Taguchi T, Nazneen A, Abid MR, Razzaque MS. 2005. "Cisplatin-associated nephrotoxicity and pathological events." *Contrib Nephrol* 148:107–21.

[95] Hoy SM. 2013. "Abiraterone acetate: a review of its use in patients with metastatic castration-resistant prostate cancer." *Drugs* 73:2077-91.

[96] Launay-Vacher V, Oudard S, Janus N, Gligorov J, Pourrat X, Rixe O, Morere JF, Beuzeboc P, Deray G; Renal Insufficiency and Cancer Medications (IRMA) Study Group. 2007. "Prevalence of Renal Insufficiency in cancer patients and implications for anticancer drug management: the renal insufficiency and anticancer medications (IRMA) study." *Cancer* 110:1376-84.

[97] Launay-Vacher V, Rey JB, Isnard-Bagnis C, Deray G, Daouphars M. 2008. "Prevention of cisplatin nephrotoxicity: state of the art and recommendations from the European Society of Clinical Pharmacy Special Interest Group on Cancer Care." *Cancer Chemother Pharmacol* 61:903-9.

[98] Filippatos TD, Milionis HJ, Elisaf MS. 2005. "Alterations in electrolyte equilibrium in patients with acute leukemia." *Eur J Haematol* 75:449–60.

[99] Yutaka Yamamoto, Yasunori Akashi, Takahumi Minami, Masahiro Nozawa, Keisuke Kiba, Motokiyo Yoshikawa, Akihide Hirayama, Hirotsugu Uemura. 2018. "Serious Hypokalemia Associated with Abiraterone Acetate in Patients with Castration-Resistant Prostate Cancer" *Case Rep Urol* 2018: 1414395.

[100] Viera AJ, Wouk N. 2015. "Potassium Disorders: Hypokalemia and Hyperkalemia." *Am Fam Physician* 92:487-95.

[101] Huang CL and Kuo E. 2007. "Mechanism of hypokalemia in magnesium deficiency". *J Am Soc Nephrol* 18:2649-52.

[102] Chakraborti S, Chakraborti T, Mandal M, Mandal A, Das S, Ghosh S. 2002. "Protective role of magnesium in the cardiovascular diseases: A review." *Mol Cell Biochem* 238 : 163 –179.

[103] Castro D, Sharma S. 2018. *Hypokalemia*. StatPearls Publishing.

[104] Kruse JA and Carlson RW. 1990. "Rapid correction of hypokalemia using concentrated intravenous potassium chloride infusions." *Arch Intern Med* 150:613–617.

[105] Agarwal A. and Wingo CS. 1999. "Treatment of hypokalemia." *N Engl J Med* 340:154–155.

[106] Asmar A, Mohandas R, Wingo CS. 2012. "A physiologic-based approach to the treatment of a patient with hypokalemia". *Am J Kidney Dis* 60:492-7.

[107] Anthony L and Vinik AI. 2011. "Evaluating the characteristics and the management of patients with neuroendocrine tumors receiving octreotide LAR during a 6-year period." *Pancreas* 40:987-94.

[108] Su H, Gu Y, Li F, Wang Q, Huang B, Jin X, Ning G, Sun F. 2013. "The PI3K/AKT/mTOR signaling pathway is overactivated in primary aldosteronism." *PLoS One* 8:e62399.

[109] Biller BM, Grossman AB, Stewart PM, Melmed S, Bertagna X, Bertherat J, Buchfelder M, Colao A, Hermus AR, Hofland LJ, Klibanski A, Lacroix A, Lindsay JR, Newell-Price J, Nieman LK, Petersenn S, Sonino N, Stalla GK, Swearingen B, Vance ML, Wass JA, Boscaro M. 2008. "Treatment of adrenocorticotropin-dependent Cushing's syndrome: a consensus statement." *J Clin Endocrinol Metab* 93:2454-62.

[110] Pessi MA, Zilembo N, Haspinger ER, Molino L, Di Cosimo S, Garassino M, Ripamonti CI. 2014. "Targeted therapy-induced diarrhea: A review of the literature." *Crit Rev Oncol Hematol* 90:165-79.

[111] Charytan D and Goldfarb DS. "Indications for hospitalization of patients with hyperkalemia." *Arch Intern Med* 160:1605-11.

[112] Su M, Stork C, Ravuri S, Lavoie T, Anguish D, Nelson LS, Hoffman RS. 2001. "Sustained-release potassium chloride overdose." *J Toxicol Clin Toxicol* 39:641-8.

[113] Nagasaki A, Takamine W, Takasu N. 2005. "Severe hyperkalemia associated with "alternative" nutritional cancer therapy." *Clin Nutr* 24:864-5.

[114] Metzner J, Evans JL, Domino KB. 2010. "Life-threatening hyperkalemia during radiofrequency ablation of hepatocellular carcinoma." *J Clin Anesth* 22:473-6.

[115] Kalemkerian GP, Darwish B, Varterasian ML. 2007. "Tumor lysis syndrome in small cell carcinoma and other solid tumors." *Am J Med* 103: 363-367.

[116] Baeksgaard L and Sorensen JB. 2003. "Acute tumor lysis syndrome in solid tumors. A case report and review of the literature." *Cancer Chemother Pharmacol* 51: 187–192.

[117] Baumann MA, Frick JC, Holoye PY. 1983. "The tumor lysis syndrome." *JAMA* 250:615.

[118] Cairo MS, Coiffier B, Reiter A, Younes A; TLS Expert Panel. 2010. "Recommendations for the evaluation of risk and prophylaxis of tumour lysis syndrome (TLS) in adults and children with malignant diseases: an expert TLS panel consensus." *Br J Haematol* 149:578-86.

[119] Liamis G, Filippatos TD, Elisaf MS. 2016. "Electrolyte disorders associated with the use of anticancer drugs." *Eur J Pharmacol* 777:78-87.

[120] Lam KY and Lo CY. 2002. "Metastatic tumours of the adrenal glands: a 30-year experience in a teaching hospital." *Clinical Endocrinology* 56.95–101.

[121] Singh N, Madan K, Aggarwal AN, Das A. 2013. "Symptomatic large bilateral adrenal metastases at presentation in small-cell lung cancer: a case report and review of the literature." *J Thorac Dis* 5:E83-6.

[122] Akcay MN, Tekin SB, Akcay G. 2003. "Addisonian crisis due to adrenal glandmetastasis in Hodgkin's disease." *International Journal of Clinical Practice* 57: 840–941.

[123] Bellevue R, Dosik H, Spergel G, Gussoff BD. 1975. "Pseudo-hyperkalemia and extreme leukocytosis." *J Lab Clin Med* 85:660–4.

[124] Mattu A, Brady WJ, Robinson DA. 2000. "Electrocardiographic manifestations of hyperkalemia." *Am J Emerg Med* 18:721-9.

[125] Kim HJ and Han SW. 2002. "Therapeutic approach to hyperkalemia." *Nephron* 92: 33–40.

[126] Maxwell AP, Linden K, O'Donnell S, Hamilton PK, McVeigh GE. 2013. "Management of hyperkalaemia." *J R Coll Physicians Edinb* 43:246-51.

[127] Sallan S. 2001. "Management of acute tumor lysis syndrome." *Semin Oncol* 28:9–12.

[128] Scott, TR., Graham, SM., Schweitzer, EJ., Bartlett, ST. 1993. "Colonic necrosis following sodium polystyrene sulphonate (Kaylexate) - sorbitol enema in a renal transplant patient: report of a case and review of the literature." *Disease of the Colon and Rectum* 36, 607–609.

[129] Watson M, Abbott KC, Yuan CM. "Damned if you do, damned if you don't: potassium binding resins in hyperkalemia." *Clin J Am Soc Nephrol.* 2010 5:1723-6.

[130] Kamel KS, Wei C. 2003. "Controversial issues in the treatment of hyperkalaemia." *Nephrol Dial Transp* 18: 2215-2218.

[131] Mahoney BA, Smith WA, Lo DS, Tsoi K, Tonelli M, Clase CM. 2005. "Emergency interventions for hyperkalaemia." *Cochrane Database Syst Rev* CD003235.

[132] Weisberg LS. 2008. "Management of severe hyperkalemia." *Crit Care Med* 36:3246-3251.

[133] Fordjour KN, Walton T, Doran JJ. 2014. "Management of hyperkalemia in hospitalized patients." *Am J Med Sci* 347:93-100.

[134] Ingram TC and Olsson JM. 2008. "In brief: hypokalemia." *Pediatr Rev* 29:e50-e51.

[135] Ngugi NN, McLigeyo SO, Kayima JK. 1997. "Treatment of hyperkalaemia by altering the transcellular gradient in patients with renal failure: effect of various therapeutic approaches." *East Afr Med* J 74:503–509.

[136] Allon M and Shanklin N. 1996. "Effect of bicarbonate administration on plasma potassium in dialysis patients: interactions with insulin and albuterol." *Am J Kidney Dis* 28:508 –514.

[137] Walser, M. 1967. "Magnesium metabolism". *Ergebnisse der Physiologie Biologischen Chemie und Experimentellen*

Pharmakologie 59: 185–296. [*Results of Physiology Biological Chemistry and Experimental Pharmacology*]

[138] Grašič Kuhar C, Strojan P, Zadnik V, Zakotnik B. 2018. "Importance of magnesium sulfate supplementation in the prevention of hypomagnesemia and hypocalcemia during chemoradiation in head and neck cancer." *J Trace Elem Med Biol* 50:327-331.

[139] Rubeiz GJ, Thill-Baharozian M, Hardie D, Carlson RW. 1993. "Association of hypomagnesemia and mortality in acutely ill medical patients." *Crit Care Med* 21:203-9.

[140] Al Ghamdi SM, Cameron EC & Sutton RA. 1994. "Magnesium deficiency: pathophysiologic and clinical overview." *American Journal of Kidney Disease* 24: 737–752.

[141] Yu ASL. 1999. Disturbances of magnesium metabolism. In: *The Kidney*. Ed: Brenner BM. WB Saunders 6th Ed, Philadelphia 1055-1070.

[142] Noronha JL and Matuschak GM. 2002. "Magnesium in critical illness: metabolism, assessment, and treatment." *Intensive Care Med* 28: 667-679.

[143] Lajer H and Daugaard G. 1999. "Cisplatin and hypomagnesemia." *Cancer Treat Rev* 25:47–58.

[144] Lajer H, Kristensen M, Hansen HH, Nielsen S, Frøkiaer J, Ostergaard LF, Christensen S, Daugaard G, Jonassen TE. 2005. "Magnesium depletion enhances cisplatin-induced nephrotoxicity". *Cancer Chemother Pharmacol* 56:535-42.

[145] Schrag D, Chung KY, Flombaum C, Saltz L. 2005. "Cetuximab therapy and symptomatic hypomagnesemia." *J. Natl. Cancer Inst.* 97:1221–1224.

[146] Wang Q, Qi Y, Zhang D, Gong C, Yao A, Xiao Y, Yang J, Zhou F, Zhou Y. 2015. "Electrolyte disorders assessment insolid tumor patients treated with anti-EGFR monoclonal antibodies: a pooled analysis of 25 randomized clinical trials." *Tumour Biol* 36,3471–3482.

[147] Vincenzi B, Santini D, Galluzzo S, Russo A, Fulfaro F, Silletta M, Battistoni F, Rocci L, Zobel BB, Adamo V, Dicuonzo G, Tonini,G. 2008. "Early magnesium reduction in advanced colorectal cancer

patients treated with cetuximab plus irinotecan as predictive factor of efficacy and outcome." *Clin. Cancer Res* 14, 4219–4224.

[148] Miltiadous G, Christidis D, Kalogirou M, Elisaf M. 2008. "Causes and mechanisms of acid-base and electrolyte abnormalities in cancer patients." *Eur J Intern Med* 19:1-7.

[149] Weisinger JR, and Bellorín-Font E. 1998. "Magnesium and phosphorus." *The Lancet* 352:391-396.

[150] Weiss-Guillet EM, Takala J, Jakob SM. 2003. "Diagnosis and management of electrolyte emergencies." *Best Pract Res Clin Endocrinol Metab* 17:623-51.

[151] Hansen BA and Bruserud Ø. 2018. "Hypomagnesemia in critically ill patients." *J Intensive Care* 6:21.

[152] Augus ZS. 1999. "Hypomagnesemia." *J Am Soc Nephrol* 10:1616-22.

[153] Morisaki H, Yamamoto S, Morita Y, Kotake Y, Ochiai R, Takeda J. 2000. "Hypermagnesemia-induced cardiopulmonary arrest before induction of anesthesia for emergency cesarean section." *J Clin Anesth* 12:224-6.

[154] Shaikh A, Berndt T, Kumar R. 2008. "Regulation of phosphate homeostasis by the phosphatonins and other novel mediators." *Pediatr Nephrol* 23:1203-10.

[155] Clinkenbeard EL and White KE. 2016. "Systemic Control of Bone Homeostasis by FGF23 Signaling." *Curr Mol Biol Rep* 2:62-71.

[156] Kalaitzidis R, Tsimihodimos V, Bairaktari E, Siamopoulos KC, Elisaf M. 2005. "Disturbances of phosphate metabolism: another feature of metabolic syndrome". *Am J Kidney Dis* 45:851-8.

[157] Yoshida T, Taguchi D, Fukuda K, Shimazu K, Inoue M, Murata K, Shibata H. 2017. "Incidence of hypophosphatemia in advanced cancer patients: a recent report from a single institution." *Int J Clin Oncol* 22:244-249.

[158] Sadot E, Zheng J, Srouji R, Strong VE, Gönen M, Balachandran VP, D'Angelica MI, Allen PJ, DeMatteo RP, Kingham TP, Fong Y, Wesier MR, Jarnagin WR. 2018. "Hypophosphatemia as a Predictor of Organ-Specific Complications Following Gastrointestinal Surgery:

Analysis of 8034 Patients." *World J Surg* doi: 10.1007/s00268-018-4726-3. [Epub ahead of print]

[159] Oronsky B, Caroen S, Oronsky A, Dobalian VE, Oronsky N, Lybeck M, Reid TR, Carter CA. 2017. "Electrolyte disorders with platinum-based chemotherapy: mechanisms, manifestations and management." *Cancer Chemother Pharmacol* 80:895-907.

[160] Berman E, Nicolaides M, Maki RG, Fleisher M, Chanel S, Scheu K, Wilson BA, Heller G, Sauter NP. 2006. "Altered bone and mineral metabolism in patients receiving imatinib mesylate." *N Engl J Med* 354:2006-13.

[161] Salomon O, Holtzman EJ, Beckerman P, Avivi C, Trakhtenbrot L, Kneller A, Tohami T, Kleinbaum Y, Apter S, Amariglio N, Grossman E, Schiby G. 2012. "Hyperphosphatemia during spontaneous tumor lysis syndrome culminate in severe hypophosphatemia at the time of blast crisis of Phneg CML to acute myelomonocytic leukemia." *Exp Hematol Oncol* 1: 24.

[162] Chong WH, Molinolo AA, Chen CC, Collins MT. 2011. "Tumor-induced osteomalacia." *Endocr Relat Cancer* 18:R53-77.

[163] Amanzadeh J and Reilly RF Jr. "Hypophosphatemia: an evidence-based approach to its clinical consequences and management." *Nat Clin Pract Nephrol* 2:136-48.

[164] Taylor BE, Huey WY, Buchman TG, Boyle WA, Coopersmith CM. 2004. "Treatment of hypophosphatemia using a protocol based on patient weight and serum phosphorus level in a surgical intensive care unit." *J Am Coll Surg* 198:198-204.

[165] Gumurdulu Y, Serin E, Ozer B, Gokcel A, Boyacioglu S. 2004. "Age as a predictor of hyperphosphatemia after oral phosphosoda administration for colon preparation." *J Gastroenterol Hepatol* 19:68-72.

[166] Howard SC, Jones DP, Pui CH. 2011. "The tumor lysis syndrome." *N Engl J Med* 364:1844-54.

[167] Hawley C. 2006. "Serum phosphate." *Nephrology* 11:S201-5.

[168] Ketteler M, Block GA, Evenepoel P, Fukagawa M, Herzog CA, McCann L, Moe SM, Shroff R, Tonelli MA, Toussaint ND, Vervloet

MG, Leonard MB. 2017. "Executive summary of the 2017 KDIGO Chronic Kidney Disease-Mineral and Bone Disorder (CKD-MBD) Guideline Update: what's changed and why it matters." *Kidney Int* 92:26-36.

[169] Hansen D, Rasmussen K, Danielsen H, Meyer-Hofmann H, Bacevicius E, Lauridsen TG, Madsen JK, Tougaard BG, Marckmann P, Thye-Roenn P, Nielsen JE, Kreiner S, Brandi L. 2011. "No difference between alfacalcidol and paricalcitol in the treatment of secondary hyperparathyroidism in hemodialysis patients: a randomized crossover trial." *Kidney Int* 80:841-50.

[170] Jones GL, Will A, Jackson GH, Webb NJ, Rule S, British Committee for Standards in Haematology. 2015. "Guidelines for the management of tumour lysis syndrome in adults and children with haematological malignancies on behalf of the British Committee for Standards in Haematology." *Br J Haematol* 169:661-71.

[171] Bailey RL, Dodd KW, Goldman JA, Gahche JJ, Dwyer JT, Moshfegh AJ, Sempos CT, Picciano MF. 2010. "Estimation of total usual calcium and vitamin D intakes in the United States." *J Nutr* 140:817-22.

[172] Ashajyothi A, Pippalla RS, Satyavati D. 2010. "Osteoporosis – An Overview." *IJPT* 2: 847-861

[173] Foley KF, Boccuzzi L. 2010. "Urine Calcium: Laboratory measurement and Clinical utility." *Lab Medicine* 41:683-686.

[174] Juppner HW, Gardella TJ, Brown EM, Kronenberg HM, Potts JT. 2001. "Parathyroid hormone and parathyroid." Jameson JL (eds) *Endocrinology*, 4th edn. Philadelphia: WB. Saunders Company : 969–998.

[175] Carney SL. 1997. "Calcitonin and human renal calcium and electrolyte transport." *Miner Electrolyte Meta* 23:43-7.

[176] DeLuca HF. 2008. "Evolution of our understanding of vitamin D". *Nutr Rev* 66:S73-87.

[177] Greco DS. 2012. "Endocrine Causes of Calcium Disorders." *Top Companion Anim Med* 27:150-5.

[178] Rizzuto R and Pozzan T. 2006. "Microdomains of intracellular Ca2+: molecular determinants and functional consequences." *Physiol Rev* 86:369-408.

[179] Bikle DD, Oda Y, Xie Z. 2004. "Calcium and 1, 25(OH)2D: interacting drivers of epidermal differentiation." *J Steroid Biochem Mol Biol* 89-90:355-60.

[180] Amuthan G, Biswas G, Ananadatheerthavarada HK, Vijayasarathy C, Shephard HM, Avadhani NG. 2002. "Mitochondrial stress-induced calcium signaling, phenotypic changes and invasive behavior in human lung carcinoma A549 cells." *Oncogene* 21:7839-49.

[181] Graber ML. 1995. "Magnesium deficiency: pathophysiologic and clinical overview." *Am J Kidney Dis* 25:973.

[182] Tohme JF and Bilezikian JP. 1993. "Hypocalcemic emergencies." *Endocrinol Metab Clin North Am* 22:363-75.

[183] Bashour T, Basha HS, Cheng TO. 1980. "Hypocalcemic cardiomyopathy." *Chest* 78:663-5.

[184] Favus MJ, Bushinsky DA, Lemann JJ. 2006. Regulation of Calcium, Magnesium, and Phosphate Metabolism. *American Society for Bone and Mineral Research Chapter* 13.

[185] Riccardi D and Brown EM. "Physiology and pathophysiology of the calcium-sensing receptor in the kidney." *Am J Physiol Renal Physiol* 298:F485-99.

[186] Zaloga GP, Willey S, Tomasic P, Chernow B. 1987. "Free fatty acids alter calcium binding: a cause for misinterpretation of serum calcium values and hypocalcemia in critical illness." *J Clin Endocrinol Metab* 64:1010-4.

[187] Inda Filho AJ and Melamed ML. 2013. "Vitamin D and Kidney disease: what we know and what we do not know." *J Bras Nefrol* 35:323-31.

[188] Campos GM, Ziemelis M, Paparodis R, Ahmed M, Davis DB. 2014. "Laparoscopic reversal of Roux-en-Y gastric bypass: technique and utility for treatment of endocrine complications." *Surg Obes Relat* Dis 10:36-43.

[189] Zhu W, Zhong M, Ai Z. 2013. "Systematic evaluation of prophylactic neck dissection for the treatment of papillary thyroid carcinoma." *Jpn J Clin Oncol* 43:883-8.

[190] Minisola S, Perugia G, Scarda A, Scarnecchia L, Tuzzolo D, Rossi W, Mazzuoli G. 1987. "Biochemical picture accompanying sclerotic bone metastases of prostatic origin." *Br J Urol* 60:443-6.

[191] Kukreja SC, Shanmugam A, Lad TE. 1988. "Hypocalcemia in patients with prostate cancer." *Calcif Tissue Int* 43:340-5.

[192] Liamis G, Milionis HJ, Elisaf M. 2009. "A review of drug-induced hypocalcemia." *J Bone Miner Metab* 27:635-42.

[193] McCormick BB, Davis J, Burns KD. 2012. "Severe hypocalcemia following denosumab injection in a hemodialysis patient." *Am J Kidney Di*s 60:626-8.

[194] Lipton A, Fizazi K, Stopeck AT, Henry DH, Brown JE, Yardley DA, Richardson GE, Siena S, Maroto P, Clemens M, Bilynskyy B, Charu V, Beuzeboc P, Rader M, Viniegra M, Saad F, Ke C, Braun A, Jun S. 2012. "Superiority of denosumab to zoledronic acid for prevention of skeletal-related events: a combined analysis of 3 pivotal, randomised, phase 3 trials." *Eur J Cancer* 48:3082-92.

[195] Fizazi K, Carducci M, Smith M, Damião R, Brown J, Karsh L, Milecki P, Shore N, Rader M, Wang H, Jiang Q, Tadros S, Dansey R, Goessl C. 2011. "Denosumab versus zoledronic acid for treatment of bone metastases in men with castration-resistant prostate cancer: a randomised, double-blind study." *Lancet* 377:813-22.

[196] Santini D, Schiavon G, Vincenzi B, Gaeta L, Pantano F, Russo A, Ortega C, Porta C, Galluzzo S, Armento G, La Verde N, Caroti C, Treilleux I, Ruggiero A, Perrone G, Addeo R, Clezardin P, Muda AO, Tonini G. 2011. "Receptor activator of NF-kB (RANK) expression in primary tumors associates with bone metastasis occurrence in breast cancer patients." *PLoS One* 6:e19234.

[197] Henry DH, Costa L, Goldwasser F, Hirsh V, Hungria V, Prausova J, Scagliotti GV, Sleeboom H, Spencer A, Vadhan-Raj S, von Moos R, Willenbacher W, Woll PJ, Wang J, Jiang Q, Jun S, Dansey R, Yeh H. 2011. "Randomized, double-blind study of denosumab versus

zoledronic acid in the treatment of bone metastases in patients with advanced cancer (excluding breast and prostate cancer) or multiple myeloma." *J Clin Oncol* 29:1125-32.

[198] Hanamura M, Iwamoto T, Soga N, Sugimura Y, Okuda M. 2010. "Risk factors contributing to the development of hypocalcemia after zoledronic acid administration in patients with bone metastases of solid tumor." *Biol Pharm Bull* 33:721-4.

[199] Milat F, Goh S, Gani LU, Suriadi C, Gillespie MT, Fuller PJ, Teede HJ, Strickland AH, Allan CA. 2013. "Prolonged hypocalcemia following denosumab therapy in metastatic hormone refractory prostate cancer". *Bone* 55:305-8.

[200] Stava CJ, Jimenez C, Vassilopoulou-Sellin R. 2007. "Endocrine sequelae of cancer and cancer treatments." *J Cancer Surviv* 1:261-74.

[201] Goren MP. 2003. "Cisplatin nephrotoxicity affects magnesium and calcium metabolism." *Med Pediatr Oncol* 41:186-9.

[202] Vandyke K, Fitter S, Dewar AL, Hughes TP, Zannettino AC. 2010. "Dysregulation of bone remodeling by imatinib mesylate." *Blood* 115:766-74.

[203] Van Vliet EI, de Herder WW, de Rijke YB, Zillikens MC, Kam BLR, Teunissen JJM, Peeters RP, Krenning EP, Kwekkeboom DJ. 2013. "Hypocalcemia after treatment with [177Lu-DOTA0,Tyr3] octreotate." *Eur J Nucl Med Mol Imaging* 40:1843-52.

[204] Qiaoli Wang, Yuexiao Qi, Di Zhang, Caifeng Gong, Anqi Yao, Yi Xiao, Jie Yang, Fuxiang Zhou, Yunfeng Zhou. 2015. "Electrolyte disorders assessment in solid tumor patients treated with anti-EGFR monoclonal antibodies: a pooled analysis of 25 randomized clinical trials." *Tumour Biol* 36: 3471–3482.

[205] Lee CT, Huynh VM, Lai LW, Lien YH. 2002. "Cyclosporine A-induced hypercalciuria in calbindin-D28k knockout and wild-type mice." *Kidney Int* 62:2055-61.

[206] Murray RM, Grill V, Crinis N, Ho PW, Davison J, Pitt P. 2001. "Hypocalcemic and normocalcemic hyperparathyroidism in patients with advanced prostatic cancer." *J Clin Endocrinol Metab* 86:4133-8.

[207] Shoback DM, Bilezikian JP, Costa AG, Dempster D, Dralle H, Khan AA, Peacock M, Raffaelli M, Silva BC, Thakker RV, Vokes T, Bouillon R. 2016. "Presentation of Hypoparathyroidism: Etiologies and Clinical Features." *J Clin Endocrinol Metab* 101:2300-12.

[208] Moore EW, Verine HJ. 1981. "Pancreatic calcification: formation constants of CaHCO3+ and CaC03(0) complexes determined with Ca2+ electrode." *Am J Physiol* 241:G182-90.

[209] Ortega B, MacWilliams JR, Dey JM, Courtright VB. 2015. "Hyperphosphatemia, hypocalcemia and increased serum potassium concentration as distinctive features of early hypomagnesemia in magnesium-deprived mice." *Magnes Res* 28:126-35.

[210] Bushinsky DA, Monk RD. 1998. "Electrolyte quintet: Calcium." *Lancet* 352:306-11.

[211] Shoback D. 2008. "Clinical practice. Hypoparathyroidism." *N Engl J Med* 359:391-403.

[212] Schafer AL, Shoback DM. "Hypocalcemia: Diagnosis and Treatment." 2016. In: De Groot LJ, Chrousos G, Dungan K, Feingold KR, Grossman A, Hershman JM, Koch C, Korbonits M, McLachlan R, New M, Purnell J, Rebar R, Singer F, Vinik A, editors. *Endotext* [Internet]. South Dartmouth (MA): MDText.com, Inc.; 2000-. Available from http://www.ncbi.nlm.nih.gov/books/NBK279022/.

[213] Trivedi DP, Doll R, Khaw KT. 2003. "Effect of four monthly oral vitamin D3 (cholecalciferol) supplementation on fractures and mortality in men and women living in the community: randomised double blind controlled trial." *BMJ* 326:469.

[214] Maeda SS, Fortes EM, Oliveira UM, Borba VC, Lazaretti-Castro M. 2006. "Hypoparathyroidism and pseudohypoparathyroidism." *Arq Bras Endocrinol Metabol* 50:664-73.

[215] Noordzij M, Voormolen NM, Boeschoten EW, Dekker FW, Bos WJ, Krediet RT, Korevaar JC; NECOSAD study group. 2009. "Disordered mineral metabolism is not a risk factor for loss of residual renal function in dialysis patients." *Nephrol Dial Transplant* 24:1580-7.

[216] Schäffler A. 2010. "Hormone replacement after thyroid and parathyroid surgery." *Dtsch Arztebl Int* 107:827-34.

[217] Brandi ML, Bilezikian JP, Shoback D, Bouillon R, Clarke BL, Thakker RV, Khan AA, Potts JT Jr. 2016. "Management of Hypoparathyroidism: Summary Statement and Guidelines." *J Clin Endocrinol Metab* 101:2273-83.

[218] Calò PG, Pisano G, Medas F, Marcialis J, Gordini L, Erdas E, Nicolosi A. 2014. "Total thyroidectomy without prophylactic central neck dissection in clinically node-negative papillary thyroid cancer: is it an adequate treatment?." *World J Surg Oncol* 12:152.

[219] Fong J, Khan A. 2012. "Hypocalcemia: updates in diagnosis and management for primary care." *Can Fam Physician* 58:158-62.

[220] Eryol NK, Colak R, Ozdoğru I, Tanriverdi F, Unal S, Topsakal R, Katlandur H, Bayram F. 2003. "Effects of calcium treatment on QT interval and QT dispersion in hypocalcemia." *Am J Cardiol* 91: 750-2.

[221] Hopper AD, Hadjivassiliou M, Butt S, Sanders DS. 2007. "Adult coeliac disease." *BMJ* 335:558-62.

[222] Bundred N. 2012. "Antiresorptive therapies in oncology and their effects on cancer progression." *Cancer Treat Rev* 38:776-86.

[223] Shepard MM, Smith JW 3rd. 2007. "Hypercalcemia." *Am J Med Sci* 334:381-5.

[224] Sava L, Pillai S, More U, Sontakke A. 2005. "Serum calcium measurement: Total versus free (ionized) calcium." *Indian J Clin Biochem* 20:158-61.

[225] Kassahun WT, Jonas S. 2011. "Focus on parathyroid carcinoma." *Int J Surg* 9:13-9.

[226] Medas F, Erdas E, Loi G, Podda F, Pisano G, Nicolosi A, Calò PG. 2016. "Controversies in the management of parathyroid carcinoma: A case series and review of the literature." *Int J Surg* 28 Suppl 1:S94-8.

[227] Hutchesson AC, Bundred NJ, Ratcliffe WA. 1995. "Survival in hypercalcaemic patients with cancer and co-existing primary hyperparathyroidism." *Postgrad Med J* 71:28-31.

[228] Saunders BD, Saunders EF, Gauger PG. 2009. "Lithium therapy and hyperparathyroidism: an evidence-based assessment." *World J Surg* 33:2314-23.

[229] Reagan P, Pani A, Rosner MH. 2014. "Approach to diagnosis and treatment of hypercalcemia in a patient with malignancy." *Am J Kidney Dis* 63:141-7.

[230] Lee CT, Yang CC, Lam KK, Kung CT, Tsai CJ, Chen HC. 2006. "Hypercalcemia in the emergency department." *Am J Med Sci* 331:119-23.

[231] Wysolmerski JJ. 2012. "Parathyroid hormone-related protein: an update." *J Clin Endocrinol Metab* 97:2947-56.

[232] Stewart AF. 2005. "Clinical practice. Hypercalcemia associated with cancer." *N Engl J Med* 352:373-9.

[233] Maarouf A, Adham M, Scoazec JY, Partensky C. 2008. "Mixed hepato/cholangiocarcinoma with paraneoplastic hypercalcemia." *J Hepatobiliary Pancreat Surg* 15:224-7.

[234] Brzozowska MM, Wolmarans L, Conaglen JV. 2009. "Hypercalcaemia caused by a carcinoid tumour." *Intern Med J* 39:415-8.

[235] Wu K, Hou SM, Huang TS, Yang RS. 2008. "Thyroid carcinoma with bone metastases: a prognostic factor study." *Clin Med Oncol* 2:129-34.

[236] Johnson RW, Nguyen MP, Padalecki SS, Grubbs BG, Merkel AR, Oyajobi BO, Matrisian LM, Mundy GR, Sterling JA. 2011. "TGF-β Promotion of Gli2-Induced Expression of Parathyroid Hormone-Related Protein, an Important Osteolytic Factor in Bone Metastasis, Is Independent of Canonical Hedgehog Signaling." *Cancer Res* 71:822-31.

[237] Giuliani N, Bataille R, Mancini C, Lazzaretti M, Barillé S. 2001. "Myeloma cells induce imbalance in the osteoprotegerin/osteoprotegerin ligand system in the human bone marrow environment." *Blood* 98:3527-33.

[238] VanHouten JN, Yu N, Rimm D, Dotto J, Arnold A, Wysolmerski JJ, Udelsman R. 2006 "Hypercalcemia of malignancy due to ectopic transactivation of the parathyroid hormone gene." *J Clin Endocrinol* Metab 91:580-3.

[239] Mirrakhimov AE. 2015. "Hypercalcemia of Malignancy: An Update on Pathogenesis and Management." *N Am J Med Sci* 7: 483–493.

[240] Liou JH, Cho LC, Hsu YH. 2006 "Paraneoplastic hypercalcemia with metastatic calcification--clinicopathologic studies." *Kaohsiung J Med* Sci 22:85-8.

[241] Stewart AF, Adler M, Byers CM, Segre GV, Broadus AE. 1982 "Calcium homeostasis in immobilization: an example of resorptive hypercalciuria." *N Engl J Med* 306:1136-40.

[242] Spinazzé S and Schrijvers D. 2006. "Metabolic emergencies." *Crit Rev Oncol Hematol* 58:79-89.

[243] Wesson LC, Suresh V, Parry RG. 2009. "Severe hypercalcaemia mimicking acute myocardial infarction." *Clin Med* (Lond) 9:186-7.

[244] Burtis CA, Ashwood ER, Bruns DE (Eds.). 2012. *Tietz textbook of clinical chemistry and molecular diagnosis* (5th Ed). Elsevier pp 1891–1965.

[245] Crowley R, Gittoes N. 2013. "How to approach hypercalcaemia." *Clin Med* (Lond) 13:287-90.

[246] Kvols LK. 2003." Neoplasms of the diffuse endocrine system". *Cancer Medicine.* Sixth Edition. Holland JF, Frei III E (Eds). Hamilton, Ontario, BC Decker, pp 1275–1323.

[247] Hagerty D R 2009. *Evidence-Based Treatment of Hypercalcemia.* Medescape. https://www.medscape.com/viewarticle/702842.

[248] Hosking DJ, Cowley A, Bucknall CA. 1981. "Rehydration in the treatment of severe hypercalcaemia". *Q J Med* 50:473-81.

[249] LeGrand SB, Leskuski D, Zama I. 2008. "Narrative review: furosemide for hypercalcemia: an unproven yet common practice." *Ann Intern Med* 149:259-63.

[250] Bilezikian JP. 1993. "Clinical review 51: Management of hypercalcemia." *J Clin Endocrinol Metab* 77:1445-9.

[251] Austin LA, Heath H 3rd. 1981. "Calcitonin: physiology and pathophysiology." *N Engl J Med* 304:269-78.

[252] Dumon JC, Magritte A, Body JJ. 1992. "Nasal human calcitonin for tumor-induced hypercalcemia." *Calcif Tissue Int* 51:18-9.

[253] Davidson TG. 2001. "Conventional treatment of hypercalcemia of malignancy." *Am J Health Syst Pharm* 58 Suppl 3:S8-15.

[254] Diskin CJ, Stokes TJ, Dansby LM, Radcliff L, Carter TB. 2007. "Malignancy-related hypercalcemia developing on a bisphosphonate but responding to calcitonin." *Clin Lung Cancer* 8:434-5.

[255] Wisneski LA. 1990. "Salmon calcitonin in the acute management of hypercalcemia." *Calcif Tissue Int* 46 Suppl:S26-30.

[256] Strumpf M, Kowalski MA, Mundy GR. 1978. "Effects of glucocorticoids on osteoclast-activating factor." *J Lab Clin Med* 92:772-8.

[257] Santini D, Vespasiani Gentilucci U, Vincenzi B, Picardi A, Vasaturo F, La Cesa A, Onori N, Scarpa S, Tonini G. 2003. "The antineoplastic role of bisphosphonates: from basic research to clinical evidence." *Ann Oncol* 14:1468-76.

[258] Xu XL, Gou WL, Wang AY, Wang Y, Guo QY, Lu Q, Lu SB, Peng J. 2013. "Basic research and clinical applications of bisphosphonates in bone disease: what have we learned over the last 40 years?" *J Transl Med* 11:303.

[259] Body JJ. 2001. "Dosing regimens and main adverse events of bisphosphonates." *Semin Oncol* 28:49-53.

[260] Gucalp R, Ritch P, Wiernik PH, Sarma PR, Keller A, Richman SP, Tauer K, Neidhart J, Mallette LE, Siegel R. 1992. "Comparative study of pamidronate disodium and etidronate disodium in the treatment of cancer-related hypercalcemia." *J Clin Oncol* 10:134-42.

[261] Nussbaum SR, Younger J, Vandepol CJ, Gagel RF, Zubler MA, Chapman R, Henderson IC, Mallette LE. 1993. "Single-dose intravenous therapy with pamidronate for the treatment of hypercalcemia of malignancy: comparison of 30-, 60-, and 90-mg dosages." *Am J Med* 95:297-304.

[262] Schwartz LM and Woloshin S. 2009. "Lost in transmission--FDA drug information that never reaches clinicians." *N Engl J Med* 361:1717-20.

[263] Liu J, Zheng L, Zhang W, Chang K, Pang Y. 2013. "A modified method for reducing renal injury in zoledronic Acid treatment of

hypercalcemia and adverse skeletal events." *Indian J Palliat Care* 19:58-63.

[264] Pecherstorfer M, Steinhauer EU, Rizzoli R, Wetterwald M, Bergström B. 2003. "Efficacy and safety of ibandronate in the treatment of hypercalcemia of malignancy: a randomized multicentric comparison to pamidronate." *Support Care Cancer* 11:539-47.

[265] Morony S, Warmington K, Adamu S, Asuncion F, Geng Z, Grisanti M, Tan HL, Capparelli C, Starnes C, Weimann B, Dunstan CR, Kostenuik PJ. 2005. "The inhibition of RANKL causes greater suppression of bone resorption and hypercalcemia compared with bisphosphonates in two models of humoral hypercalcemia of malignancy." *Endocrinology* 146:3235-43.

[266] Hanley DA, Adachi JD, Bell A, Brown V. 2012. "Denosumab: mechanism of action and clinical outcomes." *Int J Clin Pract.* 66:1139-46.

[267] Adhikaree J, Newby Y, Sundar S. 2014. "Denosumab should be the treatment of choice for bisphosphonate refractory hypercalcaemia of malignancy." *BMJ Case Rep.* pii: bcr2013202861.

[268] Cicci JD, Buie L, Bates J, van Deventer H. 2014. "Denosumab for the management of hypercalcemia of malignancy in patients with multiple myeloma and renal dysfunction." *Clin Lymphoma Myeloma Leuk* 14:e207-11.

[269] Hu MI, Glezerman IG, Leboulleux S, Insogna K, Gucalp R, Misiorowski W, Yu B, Zorsky P, Tosi D, Bessudo A, Jaccard A, Tonini G, Ying W, Braun A, Jain RK. 2014. "Denosumab for treatment of hypercalcemia of malignancy." *J Clin Endocrinol Metab* 99:3144-52.

In: New Developments in Oncology Research ISBN: 978-1-53615-365-1
Editor: Marcos T. Blair © 2019 Nova Science Publishers, Inc.

Chapter 3

ORGANODIPHOSPHINES IN $Pt\{\eta^2\text{-}P(X)_nP\}Cl_2$ (N = 5, 6, 7, 8) DERIVATIVES: STRUCTURAL ASPECTS

Milan Melník, Mária Bodnár Mikulová and Peter Mikuš
Comenius University in Bratislava, Faculty of Pharmacy,
Department of Pharmaceutical Analysis and Nuclear Pharmacy,
Bratislava, Slovak Republic
Comenius University in Bratislava, Faculty of Pharmacy,
Toxicological and Antidoping Center, Bratislava, Slovak Republic

ABSTRACT

This review includes over thirty $Pt\{\eta^2\text{-}P(X)_nP\}Cl_2$ (n = 5, 6, 7, 8) derivatives in which organodiphosphines create wide varieties of the metallocyclic rings: eight-membered (PC_5P, PC_2OC_2P, PC_2NC_2P), nine-membered (PC_6P, POC_4OP), ten-membered (POC_5OP, PC_2OCOC_2P, PC_3OC_3P), and eleven-membered (PC_8P, PNC_6NP, POC_6OP). In those derivatives the most common is a predominantly cis-arrangement (31 examples) and only 3 examples with trans-configuration. The total mean values of Pt-L bond distances in the complexes (cis- vs trans-configuration) are: 2.232 Å (L = P), 2.353 Å (L = Cl) vs 2.312 and 2.307 Å, respectively.

These data are compared and discussed with those found in cis-PtP_2Cl_2 derivatives of Pt{η^2-P(X)$_n$P}Cl_2 (n = 1,2,3,4) types. Two complexes exist in two isomeric forms cis- and trans-..

Keywords: structures, Pt{η^2-P(X)$_n$P}Cl_2 (n = 5, 6, 7, 8), review, isomers

ABBREVIATIONS

bnbp	1,1'-binaphthyl-2,2'-diyl-diphosphite
	$(C_9H_{11}O)_2P(OC_{20}H_{12}O)P(OC_9H_{11})_2$
	2,2'-bis(bis(2-isopropylphenoxy)(phosphineoxy)-1,1'-binaphthalene
(η^2-$C_{10}H_{16}O_3$)P (OC_8H_8O)P (η^2-$C_{10}H_{16}O_3$)	8,8'-(1,2-phenylenebis(methyleneoxy)bis-(1,3,5,7-tetramethyl-2,4,6-trioxa-8-phosphatricyclo[3.3.1.1^{3,7}]-decane
(η^2-$C_{16}H_{12}$)P($C_{15}H_{12}$) P(η^2-$C_{16}H_{12}$)	9,9-dimethyl-4,5-bis(2,5-diphenylphospholyl)-xanthene
(η^2-$C_{20}H_{12}O_2$) P($C_{15}H_{12}O$) P(η^2-$C_{20}H_{12}O_2$)	4,5-bis(dinaphtho[2,1-d:1',2'-f][1,3,2]-dioxa-phosphin)-9,9-dimethylxantene
(η^2-$C_{22}H_{28}O_3$) P($C_{15}H_{12}O$) P(η^2-$C_{22}H_{28}O_3$)	4,5-bis(3-terc-butyl-5-methoxy-1,1'-biphenyl-2,2'-dioxy)phosphino-9,9-dimethylxantene
(η^2-C_8H_{12})P($C_{14}H_{16}$) P(η^2-C_8H_{12})	2,2'-bis((9-phosphabicyclo[3.3.1]nonan-9-yl)-methyl)-1,1'-biphenyl
$Ph_2P(C1_{18}H_{12})PPh_2$	1,2-bis(2-(diphenylphosphino)phenyl)benzene

$Ph_2P(C_{13}H_8O)PPh_2$	2,2'-bis(diphenylphosphino)benzophenone
$Ph_2P(C_{14}H_{12}OSi)PPh_2$	4,6-bis(diphenylphosphino)-10,10-dimethyl-10H-phenoxasilin
$Ph_2P(C_{16}H_{12}O)PPh_2$	bis(diphenylphosphino)-9,9-dimethyl-9H-xanthene-4,5-diyl
$Ph_2P(C_{16}H_{14})PPh_2$	tricyclo[8.2.2.2^4]hexadeca-1(12)-4,6,10,13,15-hexane-5,12-diyl-bis(diphenylphosphane)
$Ph_2P(C_{20}H_{12})PPh_2$	1,8-bis(diphenylphosphino)triptycene
$Ph_2P(C_{20}H_{16}O_2)PPh_2$	1,2-bis(3-(diphenylphosphino)-4-methoxyphenyl)benzene
$Ph_2P(C_{23}H_{26}O_2)PPh_2$	8,8'-bis(diphenylphosphido)-4,4,4',4',6,6'-hexamethylspiro-2,2'-bichroman
$Ph_2P(C_6H_8O_3)PPh_2$	3,6-bis(diphenylphosphinooxy)-hexahydrofuro-(3,2-b)furan
$Ph_2P(C_7H_6OC_7H_6O)$ PPh_2	((oxy(bis)methylene-2,1-phenylene))bis(diphenyl-phosphine)
$Ph_2P(CH_2)_5PPh_2$	1,5-bis(diphenylphosphino)pentane
$Ph_2P(NC_{12}H_8N)PPh_2$	5,10-bis(diphenylphosphino)phenozine
$Ph_2P(OC_7H_{10}O)PPh_2$	(3-endo-6-endo-bis(diphenylphosphinooxy) bicyclo[3.2.0]-heptane)
$Ph_2P\{(CH_2)_2N(P)$ $(CH_2)_2P\}PPh_2$	N,N-bis(2-(diphenylphosphino)ethyl)aniline
$Ph_2P\{C_{10}H_6(CH_2)$ $C_{10}H_6O\}PPh_2$	1,1'-methylene-bis(2-((diphenylphosphino)oxy)-naphthalene
$Ph_2P\{OC_6H_4(CH_2)$ $C_6H_4O\}PPh_2$	methylene-di-2,1-phenylenebis(diphenylphosphinate)
$Pr^i_2P(C_{18}H_{24})PPr^i_2$	([1^1,2^1:2^2,3^1-terphenyl]-1^2,3^2-diyl)-[bis(bis(propan-2-yl)-phosphane]
$Pr^i_2P(C_{20}H_{12})PPr^i_2$	1,8-bis(diisopropylphosphino)triptycene
$Pr^i_2P(OC_{12}H_8O)PPr^i_2$	2,2'-bis(diisopropylphosphinito)-1,1'-biphenyl
$Pr^i_2P(OC_{14}H_{12}O)PPr^i_2$	2,2'-bis(diisopropylphosphanyloxymethyl)-1,1'-biphenyl

$Pr^i_2P(OC_6H_{10}O)PPr^i_2$	1,3-bis(diisopropylphosphonite)cyclohexane
$Pr^i_2P\{OC_{12}H_8(CH_2)O\}PPr^i_2$	(2-diisopropylphosphanyloxy-2'-diisopropyl-phosphanyloxymethyl-1,1'-biphenyl

1. Introduction

Platinum chemistry is very attractive and useful. Organodiphosphines as soft donor ligands are often present in platinum complexes. Recently we classified and analyzed structural parameters of organodiphosphines as chelating ligands in PtP_2Cl_2 derivatives. On the basis of the coordination mode of the respective chelating ligands there are complexes in which the chelating ligands create four- and five-membered metallocyclic rings [1], six-membered [2] and seven-membered [3].

The aim of this review is classify and analyze structural parameters of monomeric $Pt\{\eta^2\text{-}P(X)_nP\}Cl_2$ (n = 5, 6, 7, 8) in which organodiphosphines create eight- nine- ten- and eleven-membered metallocyclic rings.

2. $Pt\{\eta^2\text{-}P(X)_nP\}Cl_2$ (n = 5, 6, 7, 8) Derivatives

There are over thirty examples of monomeric Pt(II) complexes in which chelating organodiphosphines create: eight-, nine-, ten-, and eleven-membered metallocyclic rings.

2.1. Cis- $Pt\{\eta^2\text{-}P(X)_5P\}Cl_2$ Type

There are thirteen complexes in which organodiphosphine ligands create eight-membered metallocyclic rings and a pair of chlorides completed a square-planar environment about each Pt(II) atom with various degrees of distortion. These complexes crystallize in three crystal systems: triclinic (2 examples), monoclinic (5 examples) and orthorhombic (6 examples). In five complexes, namely: $[Pt\{\eta^2\text{-}Ph_2P(CH_2)_5PPh_2\}(Cl)_2]$ [4], $[Pt\{\eta^2\text{-}Ph_2P(C_{13}H_8O)PPh_2\}(Cl)_2].2CH_2Cl_2$ (at 100K) [5], $[Pt\{\eta^2\text{-}Pr^i{}_2P(C_{20}H_{12})PPr^i{}_2\}(Cl)_2].2CHCl_3$ (at 173K) [6], $[Pt\{\eta^2\text{-}Ph_2P(C_{20}H_{12})PPh_2\}(Cl)_2]$ (at 150K) [7], and $[Pt\{\eta^2\text{-}Ph_2P(C_{12}H_{10})PPh_2\}(Cl)_2]$. CH_2Cl_2 [8], the respective chelating organodiphosphine ligands create eight- membered metallocyclic rings (PC_5P) with the mean value of P-Pt-P bite angles of 102.2°.

In another five complexes: $[Pt\{\eta^2\text{-}Ph_2P(C_{16}H_{12}O)PPh_2\}(Cl)_2]$. $3.25CH_2Cl_2$ [9], $[Pt\{\eta^2\text{-}Ph_2P(C_{14}H_{12}OSi)PPh_2\}(Cl)_2]MeCN$ (at 150K) [10], $[Pt\{\eta^2\text{-}(\eta^2\text{-}C_{20}H_{12}O_2)P(C_{15}H_{12}O)P(\eta^2\text{-}C_{20}H_{12}O_2)\}(Cl)_2].MeCN.CH_2Cl_2$ (at 150K) [11], $[Pt\{\eta^2\text{-}(\eta^2\text{-}C_{22}H_{28}O_3)P(C_{15}H_{12}O)P(\eta^2\text{-}C_{22}H_{28}O_3)\}(Cl)_2]$ (at 150K) [12], and $[Pt\{\eta^2\text{-}(\eta^2\text{-}C_{16}H_{12})P(C_{15}H_{12})P(\eta^2\text{-}C_{16}H_{12})\}(Cl)_2].CH_2Cl_2$ (at 150K) [13] the chelating organodiphosphine ligands form eight-membered metallocyclic rings (PC_2OC_2P) with the mean value of the P-Pt-P bite angles of 100.9°. Structure of $[Pt\{\eta^2\text{-}Ph_2P(C_{14}H_{12}OSi)PPh_2\}(Cl)_2]$ [10] is shown in Figure 1 as an example.

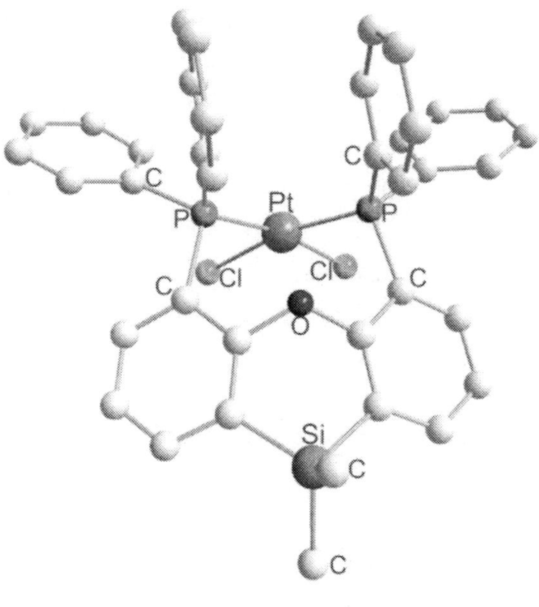

Figure 1. Structure of $[Pt\{\eta^2\text{-}Ph_2P(C_{14}H_{12}OSi)PPh_2\}(Cl)_2]$ [10].

In $[Pt\{\eta^2\text{-}Pr^i_2P(OC_6H_{10}O)PPr^i_2\}(Cl)_2]$ (at 150K) ([14], the chelating P,P-donor ligand creates an eight-membered metallocyclic ring (POC_3OP) with the value of P-Pt-P bite angle of 100.2°. In $[Pt\{\eta^2\text{-}Ph_2P(CH_2)_2N(Ph)(CH_2)_2PPh_2\}(Cl)_2].CH_2Cl_2$ (at 170K) [15], the chelating P,P-donor ligand creates eight-membered metallocyclic ring (PC_2NC_2P) with the value of P-Pt-P bite angle of 101.0°. In $[Pt\{\eta^2\text{-}Pr^i_2P\{N(H)N(Me)P(S)(Ph)N(Me)N(H)\}PPr^i_2](Cl)_2$ [16], the chelating P,P-donor ligand creates PN_2PN_2P ring (100.6°).

In these complexes the total mean values of cis-L-Pt-L bond angles open in the sequence: 85.7° (Cl-Pt-P) < 86.4° (Cl-Pt-Cl) < 101.3° (P-Pt-P), and the mean value of trans-Cl-Pt-P bond angles is 172.5°. The total mean value of Pt-L bond distances is 2.248 Å (range 2.235 – 2.262 Å) (L=P) and 2.354 Å (range 2.342 – 2.362 Å) (L=Cl).

2.2. Cis-$Pt\{\eta^2\text{-}P(X)_6P\}Cl_2$ Type

There are nine examples in which chelating organodiphosphine ligands create nine- membered metallocyclic rings. These complexes crystallize in two crystal systems: triclinic (4 examples) and monoclinic (5 examples). On the basis of the respective metallocyclic rings these complexes can be divided into the two sub-groups. In the following four complexes: $[Pt\{\eta^2\text{-}bnbp\}(Cl)_2]$ [17], $[Pt\{\eta^2\text{-}Ph_2P(C_{18}H_{12})PPh_2\}(Cl)_2]$ [18], $[Pt\{\eta^2\text{-}Pr^i_2P(C_{18}H_{24})PPr^i_2\}(Cl)_2]$. C_6H_6 (at 120K) [19], (Figure 2) and $[Pt\{\eta^2\text{-}(\eta^2\text{-}C_8H_{12})P(C_{14}H_{16})P(\eta^2\text{-}C_8H_{12})\}(Cl)_2]$ [20] the chelating orgnodiphosphine ligands create nine-membered metallocyclic rings (PC_6P) with the mean value P-Pt-P bite angles of 95.0°.

In the remaining five complexes: $[Pt\{\eta^2\text{-}Ph_2P(OC_7H_{10}O)PPh_2\}(Cl)_2].2CH_2Cl_2$ (at 115K) [21], $[Pt\{\eta^2\text{-}Pr^i_2P(OC_{12}H_8O)PPr^i_2\}(Cl)_2]$ (at 123K) [22], $[Pt\{\eta^2\text{-}Ph_2P(OC_{12}H_8O)PPh_2\}(Cl)_2]CH_2Cl_2$ (at 173K) [22], $[Pt\{\eta^2\text{-}(\eta^2\text{-}C_{10}H_{16}O_3)P(OC_8H_8O)P(\eta^2\text{-}C_{10}H_{16}O_3)\}(Cl)_2].CH_2Cl_2$ (at 100K) [23], and $[Pt\{\eta^2\text{-}(C_9H_{11}O)_2P(OC_{20}H_{12}O)P(OC_9H_{11})_2\}(Cl)_2].0.35CH_2Cl_2$. 2.3MeCN (at 125K) [24], each chelating organodiphosphine ligand creates nine-membered metallocyclic ring (POC_4OP) with mean value of P-Pt-P bite angles of 95.4°. In this series of complexes the cis-L-Pt-P bond angles (mean values) open in the sequence: 86.7° (Cl-Pt-Cl) < 89.0° (Cl-Pt-P) < 95.3° (P-Pt-P). The mean value of trans-Cl-Pt-P bond angles is 173.5°. The total mean values of Pt-L bond distances are: 2.205 (range 2.185 – 2.220 Å) (L = P) and 2.335 (range 2.323 – 2.355 Å (L = Cl).

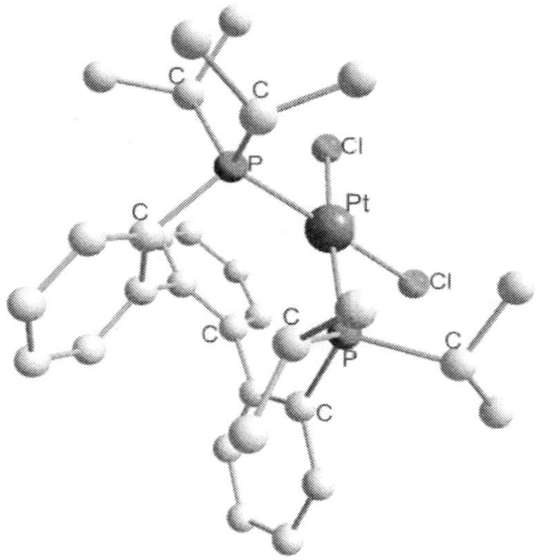

Figure 2. Structure of [Pt{η^2-$Pr^i_2P(C_{18}H_{24})PPr^i_2$}$(Cl)_2$] [19].

2.3. Cis- and Trans-Pt{η^2-$P(X)_7P$}Cl_2 Type

In two monoclinic cis-complexes [Pt{η^2-Ph_2P{$OC_{10}H_6(CH_2)C_{10}H_6O$}$PPh_2$}$(Cl)_2$].$CH_2Cl_2.H_2O$ [25], and [Pt{η^2-Ph_2P{$OC_6H_4(CH)_2C_6H_4O$}$PPh_2(Cl)_2$].CH_2Cl_2 (at 103K) [26] the chelating organodiphosphine ligands create ten-membered metallocyclic rings of the composition (POC_5OP) with the mean values of P-Pt-P bite angles of 95.5° and Cl-Pt-Cl of 89.1°. The mean Pt-P and Pt-Cl bond distances are 2.231 and 2.356 Å, respectively.

A similar ring (POC_5OP) was found in monoclinic cis- and triclinic trans-[Pt{η^2-Pr^i_2P{$OC_{12}H_8(CH_2)O$}PPr^i_2}$(Cl)_2$].$2CHCl_3$ (at 173K) [27]. Structure of the cis-isomers is shown in Figure 3. In the cis-isomer the values of P-Pt-P and Cl-Pt-Cl bond angles are 95.9 and 85.6°, respectively. The mean values of Pt-L bond distances are 2.247 Å (L = P) and 2.358 Å (L = Cl), respectively. The trans-isomer contains two crystallographically independent molecules. In trans-isomer the values of trans-P-Pt-P and trans-Cl-Pt-Cl bond angles (molecule 1 vs molecule 2) are 171.5 and 178.4° vs 170.3 and 177.8°. The mean values of Pt-L bond distances are 2.309 Å (L = P) and 2.307 Å (L = Cl) in molecule 1 and in molecule 2 the values are 2.314 and 2.306 Å, respectively. The Pt-Cl bond distance in the cis-isomer of 2.358 Å is longer than that in the trans-isomer (2.307 Å) as a reason of higher trans-influence of P over Cl. The sum of all four (Pt-P(x2) + Pt-Cl(x2)) bond distances growing in the order: 9.121 Å (cis- isomer) < 9.232 (trans-molecule 1) < 9.240 Å (trans-molecule 2). This indicates that in the given order the covalent bond is somewhat weakness (Pt-L).

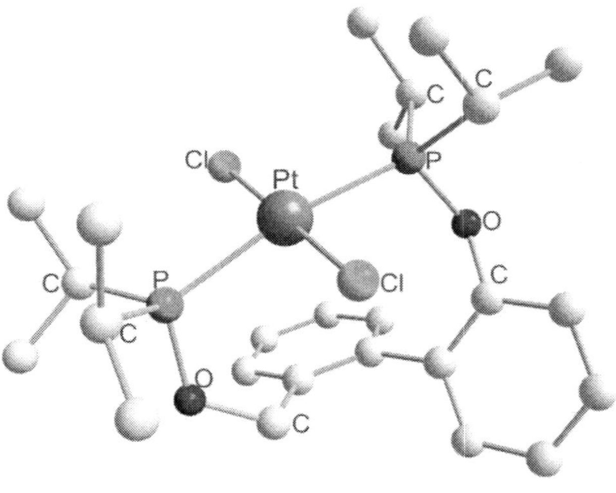

Figure 3. Structure of cis-[Pt{η^2-Pr^i_2P{$OC_{12}H_8(CH_2)O$}PPr^i_2}$(Cl)_2$] [27].

In orthorhombic cis-[Pt{η^2-$Ph_2P(C_{23}H_{26}O_2)PPh_2$}$(Cl)_2$] [28] the chelating ligand creates ten-membered metallocyclic ring (PC_2OCOC_2P) with the value of P-Pt-P bite angle of 96°. In monoclinic cis-[Pt{η^2-$Ph_2P(C_6H_8O_3)PPh_2$}$(Cl)_2$] [29] the organodiphosphine ligand forms (POC_2OC_2OP) ring with the value of P-Pt-P bond angle of 96.2°. In triclinic cis-[Pt{η^2-$Ph_2P(C_7H_6OC_7H_6)PPh_2$}$(Cl)_2$].$CH_2Cl_2$ (at 100K) [30] the organodiphosphine ligand creates ten-membered metallocyclic ring (PC_3OC_3P) with P-Pt-P bite angle of 96.5°.

In this series of cis- complexes the cis-L-Pt-L bond angles (mean values) open in the sequence: 87.4° (Cl-Pt-Cl) < 88.5° (Cl-Pt-P) < 95.7° (P-Pt-P). The mean values of Pt-L bond distances are 2.239 (range 2.29 – 2.253) Å (L = P) and 2.354 (range 2.229 – 2.253) Å (L = Cl).

2.4. Cis- and Trans-Pt{η^2-P(X)$_8$P)Cl$_2$ Type

In two monoclinic cis-complexes: [Pt{η^2-$Ph_2P(C_{20}H_{16}O_2)PPh_2$}$(Cl)_2$].$CDCl_3$ (at 100K) [18], and [Pt{η^2-$Ph_2P(C_{16}H_{14})PPh_2$}$(Cl)_2$] (at 150K) (Figure 4) [31] organodiphosphine ligands create eleven-membered metallocyclic rings (PC_8P) with the mean P-Pt-P bite angles of 97.0°. In another monoclinic cis-[Pt{η^2-$Ph_2P(NC_{12}H_8N)PPh_2$}$(Cl)_2$] (at 125K) [32] the chelating P,P-donor ligand creates (PNC_6NP) metallocyclic ring (97.6°).

Monoclinic [Pt{η^2-$Pr^i_2P(OC_{14}H_{12}O)PPr^i_2$}$(Cl)_2$] (at 173K) [27] exists in two isomeric forms: cis- (contains 3$CHCl_3$ solvate) and trans. In both isomers the chelating ligand creates POC_6OP-metallocyclic rings with the values of P-Pt-P bite angles of 96.6° (cis-isomer) and 177.9° (trans-isomer). In cis-isomer the mean values of Pt-P and Pt-Cl bond distances are 2.237 and 2.376 Å and Cl-Pt-Cl bond angle is 85.4°. In trans-isomer the values are 2.323 and 2.305 Å. The value of trans-Cl-Pt-Cl bond angle is 173.5°.

In this series of cis-complexes the total mean values of cis-L-Pt-L bond angles are 97.0° (P-Pt-P) and 86.0° (Cl-Pt-Cl). The total mean values of Pt-L bond distances are 2.237 Å (L = P) and 2.370 Å (L = Cl). In trans-derivative the mean values of trans-L-Pt-L bond angles are 176.2° (P-Pt-P) and 173.2° (Cl-Pt-Cl). The mean values of Pt-L bond distances are 2.320 Å (L = P) and 2.303 Å (L = Cl).

There are 31 examples with cis-configuration and 3 examples with trans-configuration. The total mean values of Pt-L bond distances in the complexes (cis- vs trans-configuration) are 2.232 Å (L = P), 2.353 Å (L = Cl) vs 2.312 and 2.307 Å, respectively.

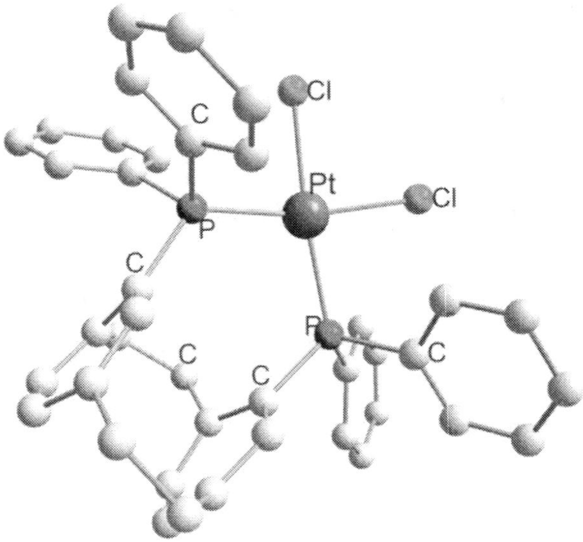

Figure 4. Structure of [Pt{η^2-$Ph_2P(C_{16}H_{14})PPh_2$}$(Cl)_2$] [31].

Conclusion

This review covers over thirty monomeric complexes of Pt{η^2-$P(X)_nP$}Cl_2 (n = 5,6,7,8) type. The chelating organodiphosphine ligands create eight-, nine-, ten-, and eleven-membered metallocyclic rings. These complexes crystalize in three crystal systems: orthorhombic (6 examples), triclinic (8 examples) and monoclinic (20 examples). In cis-Pt{η^2-$P(X)_5P$}Cl_2 type, the chelating P,P-donor ligands create the following eight-membered metallocyclic rings: PC_5P (5 examples), PC_2OC_2P (5 examples), PC_2NC_2P (1 example), and POC_3OP (1 example). The cis-L-Pt-L bond angles (total mean values) open in the sequence: 85.7° (Cl-Pt-P) < 86.4° (Cl-Pt-Cl) < 101.3° (P-Pt-P). The value of trans-Cl-Pt-P bond angles is 172.5°. The Pt-L bond distances (total mean values) are 2.248 Å (L = P) and 2.354 Å (L = Cl).

In cis-Pt{η^2-$P(X_6)P$}Cl_2 type the chelating ligands create the following nine-membered metallocyclic rings: P (4 example) and POC_4OP (5 examples). The cis-L-Pt-L bond angles (total mean values) open in the sequence: 86.7° (Cl-Pt-Cl) < 89.0° (Cl-Pt-P) < 95.3° (P-Pt-P). The mean value of trans-Cl-Pt-P bond angles is 173.5°.

In cis-Pt{η^2-P(X)$_7$P}Cl$_2$ type the chelating ligands form the following ten-membered metallocyclic rings: POC$_5$OP (3 examples), POC$_2$OC$_2$OP (1 example), PC$_2$OCOC$_2$P (1 example) and PC$_3$OC$_3$P (1 example). The cis-L-Pt-L bond angles, (total mean values) open in the order: 86.7° (Cl-Pt-Cl) < 88.5° (Cl-Pt-P) < 95.7° (P-Pt-P). The mean value of trans-Cl-Pt-P bond distances are 2.239 Å (L = P) and 2.354 Å (L = Cl).

In cis-Pt{η^2-P(X)$_8$P}Cl$_2$ type, the chelating ligands create the following metallocyclic rings: PC$_8$P (2 examples), PNC$_6$NP (1 example), and POC$_6$OP (1 example). The cis-L-Pt-L bond angles (total mean values) open in the sequence: 86.0° (Cl-Pt-Cl) < 88.4° (Cl-Pt-P) < 97.3° (P-Pt-P). The mean value of trans-Cl-Pt-P bond angles is 175.0°. The mean values of Pt-L bond distances are 2.237 Å (L = P) and 2.370 Å (L = Cl).

The [Pt{η^2-Pr$^i_2$P{OC$_{12}$H$_8$(CH$_2$)O}PPr$^i_2$}(Cl)$_2$] [27] exists in two isomeric forms: monoclinic cis- and triclinic trans. The trans-isomer contains two crystallographically independent molecules differ mostly by degree of distortion. These complexes belong to the unusual combination of isomerism, cis-, trans- and distortion [33]. Monoclinic [Pt{η^2-Pr$^i_2$P{OC$_{14}$H$_{12}$)PPr$^i_2$}(Cl)$_2$] [27] exists in two isomeric forms cis- and trans.

Organodiphosphines as soft donor chelating ligands is very attractive and useful especially in the chemistry of platinum. There are more than 180 monomeric platinum complexes of the Pt{η^2-P$_2$L)Cl$_2$ type which were studied by X-ray analyze. Selected structural data of the complexes with cis-configuration are summarized in Table 1.

There are at least two contributing factors to the size of the P-Pt-P bond angles, both ligands based. One is the steric constraints imposed on the ligand and the other is the need to accommodate bidenticity there appropriate.

Comparing the bidentate P-Pt-P angles it is seen that in there is an increase in value as the size from four- to eight-membered of the metallocyclic ring increases parallels an increase in Pt-P bond distance and at the same time the value of cis-Cl-Pt-Cl and cis-Cl-Pt-P angles decrease. No such trends were found for the complexes with nine-, ten-, and eleven-membered metallocyclic rings. One of the reasons can be "twist" of the respective metallocycles.

Table 1. The total mean values of selected structural parameters of Pt{η^2-P_2L)Cl_2 Derivatives

Metallocyclic ring (number of examples)	P-Pt-P [°]	Cl-Pt-Cl [°]	Cl-Pt-P [°]	Pt-P [Å]	Pt-Cl [Å]	∑Pt-L(x4) [Å]
four-membered [1] (24)	72.4	91.7	97.3 170.4	2.214	2.352	9.13
five-membered [1] (51)	86.4	88.0	92.7 175.7	2.216	2.354	9.14
six-membered [2] (42)	94.0	87.6	89.0 175.6	2.222	2.358	9.16
seven-membered [3] (34)	96.8	87.2	87.7 173.5	2.239	2.350	9.17
eight-membered[a] (12)	101.3	86.4	85.7 172.5	2.248	2.354	9.20
nine-membered[a] (9)	95.0	86.7	89.0 173.5	2.205	2.335	9.08
ten-membered[a] (7)	95.7	87.4	88.5 174.0	2.239	2.354	9.18
eleven-membered[a] (6)	97.3	86.0	88.4 175.0	2.237	2.370	9.21

[a.] This work.

The mean Pt-Cl and Pt-P bob distances at 2.353 Å and 2.232 Å respectively for cis and 2.307 and 2.312 Å respectively for trans. The cis-derivatives tend to be more crowded than the trans-derivatives as seen by comparing the sum of the Pt-L bond distances at 9.17 Å and 9.25 Å respectively.

During the collection and organization of the data has become evident that some original papers are lacking important information such as atomic coordinates and analysis of intermolecular distances. In view of these limitations we believe that a review such as this can continue to serve a useful function by centralizing available material and delineating areas worthy of further investigation

ACKNOWLEDGMENTS

This work was supported by the projects VEGA 1/0463/18, and APVV-15-0585.

REFERENCES

[1] Melník M., Forgácsová A., Mikuš P. Organodiphosphines in cis-Pt(η^2-PXP)Cl_2 and Pt(η^2-PXXP)Cl_2 derivatives: structural aspects, *New Developments in Oncology Research*, Nova Science Publ. Inc., NY, USA, 2018, Chapter 1.

[2] Melník M., Forgácsová A., Mikuš P. Organodiphosphines in cis-Pt(η^2-PXXP)Cl_2 derivatives – structural aspects, *New Developments in Oncology Research*, Nova Science Publ. Inc., NY, USA, 2018, Chapter 2.

[3] Melník M., Forgácsová A., Mikuš P. Organodiphosphines in Pt(η^2-PXXXXP)Cl_2 derivatives – structural aspects, *New Developments in Oncology Research*, Nova Science Publ. Inc., NY, USA, 2018, Chapter 3.

[4] Klein H. P., Thewalt U., Zettlmeissl H., Brune H. A., *cis*-Dichloro-(1,5-bisdiphenylphosphanopentan)platin(II). Synthese, Kristall- und Molekulstruktur, *Z. Naturforsch.*, 1981, 36b, 1125-1129.

[5] Mikami K., Wakabayashi K., Yusa Y., Aikawa K., Achiral benzophenone ligand–rhodium complex with chiral diamine activator for high enantiocontrol in asymmetric transfer hydrogenation, *Chem. Commun.*, 2006, 2365-2367.

[6] Azerraf C., Grossman O., Gelman D., Rigid *trans*-spanning triptycene-based ligands: How flexible they can be?, *J. Organomet. Chem.*, 2007, 692, 761-767.

[7] Bini L., Muller C., Wilting J., von Chrzanowski L., Spek A. L., Vogt D., Highly Selective Hydrocyanation of Butadiene toward 3-Pentenenitrile, *J. Am. Chem. Soc.*, 2007, 129, 12622-12623.

[8] Yamamoto Y., Fukui Y., Matsubara K., Takeshima H., Miyauchi F., Tanase T., Yamamoto G., Preparation and characterization of palladium and platinum complexes bearing 1,8-bis[(diphenyl phosphino)methyl]naphthalene, *J. Chem. Soc., Dalton Trans.*, 2001, 1773-1781.

[9] Niksch T., Gorls H., Friedrich M., Oilunkaniemi R., Laitinen R., Weigand W., Synthesis and Characterisation of 2,2-Bis (hydroxymethyl)-1,3-diselenolato Metal(II) Complexes Bearing Various Phosphanes, *Eur. J. Inorg. Chem.*, 2010, 74-94.

[10] van Duren R., van der Vlugt J. I, Kooijman H., Spek A. L., Vogt D., Platinum-catalyzed hydroformylation of terminal and internal octenes, *Dalton Trans.*, 2007, 1053-1059.

[11] van Duren R., Cornelissen L. J. M., van der Vlugt J. I., Huijbers J. P. J., Mills A. M., Spek A. L., Muller C., Vogt D., Chiral (Diphosphonite)platinum Complexes in Asymmetric Hydroformylation, *Helv. Chim. Acta*, 2006, 89, 1547-1558.

[12] van der Vlugt J. I., Sablong R., Mills A. M., Kooijman H., Spek A. L., Meetsma A., Vogt D., *Coordination chemistry and X-ray studies with novel sterically constrained diphosphonite ligands*, Dalton Trans., 2003, 4690-4699.

[13] Mora G., Piechaczyk O., Houdard R., Mezailles N., Le Goff X. F., Le Floch P., Why Platinum Catalysts Involving Ligands with Large Bite Angle Are so Efficient in the Allylation of Amines: Design of a Highly Active Catalyst and Comprehensive Experimental and DFT Study, *Chem. Eur. J,* 2008, 14, 10047-10057.

[14] Olsson D., Arunachalampillai A., Wendt O. F., Synthesis and characterisation of $PC_{sp3}P$ phosphine and phosphinite platinum(II) complexes. Cyclometallation and simple coordination, *Dalton Trans.*, 2007, 5427-5433.

[15] Kostas I. D., Antonopoulou G., Potamitis C., Raptopoulou C. P., Psycharis V., Platinum complexes with a methoxy-amino phosphine or a nitrogen-containing bis(phosphine) ligand. Synthesis, characterization and application to hydrogenation of trans-cinnamaldehyde, *J. Organomet. Chem.,* 2017, 828, 133-141.

[16] Sreenivasa Reddy V., Katti K. V., Barnes C. L., Transition Metal Chemistry of Main Group Hydrazides. 8. A new Long-Chain Diphosphine with the P^{III}-N-N-P^{V}-N-N-P^{III} Backbond as a Chelating Ligand for Molybdenum, Platinum, and Palladium. Crystal and Molecular Structures of *cis*-[Mo(CO)$_4${PhP(S)[N(Me)NHP(*i*-Pr)$_2$]$_2$}] and *cis*-[PtCl$_2${PhP(S)[N(Me)NHP(*i*-Pr)$_2$]$_2$}], *Organometallics*, 1994, 13, 2391-2396.

[17] Nifant′ev E. E., Rasadkina E. N., Batalova T. A., Bekker A. R., Stash A.I., Belskii V.K., Crystal and molecular structure of bis(1,1′-binaphthyl-2,2′-diyl-diphosphite)dichloro-platinum(II) complex, Zh. *Obsch. Khim*., 1996, 66, 1109-1112.

[18] van der Vlugt J. I., van Duren R., Batema G. D., den Heeten R., Meetsma A., Fraanje J., Goubitz K., Kamer P. C. J., van Leeuwen P., Vogt D., Platinum Complexes of Rigid Bidentate Phosphine Ligands in the Hydroformylation of 1-Octene, *Organometallics,* 2005, 24, 5377-5382.

[19] Barrett B. J., Iluc V. M., An Adaptable Chelating Diphosphine Ligand for the Stabilization of Palladium and Platinum Carbenes, *Organometallics,* 2017, 36, 730-741.

[20] Eberhard M. R., Heslop K. M., Orpen A. G., Pringle P. G., Nine-Membered Trans Square-Planar Chelates Formed by a bisbi Analogue, *Organometallics*, 2005, 24, 335-337.

[21] Fairlamb I. J. S., Grant S., Whitwood A. C., Whitthall J., Batsanov A. S., Collings J. C., Synthesis of Pd(II) and Pt(II) complexes possessing bicyclo[3.2.0]heptanyl phosphinite ligands: Identification of a novel Pd(II) precatalyst for 1,6-diene cycloisomerisation, *J. Organomet. Chem.,* 2005, 690, 4462-4477.

[22] Ruhland K., Herdtweck E., Mechanistic investigation of the thermal decomposition of Biphen (OP*i*-Pr) PtEt$_2$: An entrance into C–C single bond activation*?, J. Organomet. Chem*., 2005, 690, 5215-5236.

[23] Mikhel I. S., Garland M., Hopewell J., Mastroianni S., McMullin C. L., Orpen A. G., Pringle P. G., Cage Phosphinites: Ligands for Efficient Nickel-Catalyzed Hydrocyanation of 3-Pentenenitrile, *Organometallics,* 2011, 30, 974-985.

[24] Wilting J., Janssen M., Muller C., Lutz M., Spek A. L., Vogt D., Binaphthol-Based Diphosphite Ligands in Asymmetric Nickel-Catalyzed Hydrocyanation of Styrene and 1,3-Cyclohexadiene: Influence of Steric Properties, *Adv. Synth. Catal.*, 2007, 349, 350-356.

[25] Balakrishna M. S., Panda R., Mague J. T., Synthesis and derivatization, structures and transition metal chemistry of a new large bite bis(phosphinite) derived from bis(2-hydroxy-1-naphthyl) methane, *J. Chem. Soc., Dalton Trans.*, 2002, 4617-4621.

[26] Irisli S., Guzelsoylu C., Karaman M., Buyukgungor O., Chelated palladium and platinum complexes of diphosphinite ligands, ch_2(o-$c_6h_4$opph$_2$)$_2$ and ph$_2$po(ch$_2$)$_3$opph$_2$: characterization and catalytic activity, *Phosphorus, Sulfur, Silicone, Relat. Elem.*, 2015, 190, 1668-1679.

[27] Ruhland K., Bruck A., Herdtweck E., Investigation of the Thermal Decomposition of [biphen(QP*i*Pr)Pt(alk)$_2$]: An Entry to C–C Single Bond Activation?, *Eur. J. Inorg. Chem.*, 2007, 944-964.

[28] Freixa Z., Beentjes M. S., Batema G. D., Dieleman C. B., van Strijdonck G. P. F., Reek J. N. H., Kamer P. C. J., Fraanje J., Goubitz K., van Leeuwen P. W. N. M., SPANphos: A C_2-Symmetric *trans*-Coordinating Diphosphane Ligand, *Angew. Chem., Int.* Ed., 2003, 42, 1284-1287.

[29] Sharma R. K., Samuelson A. G., Asymmetric allylation of aldehydes with chiral platinum phosphinite complexes, *Tetrahedron: Asymm.*, 2007, 18, 2387-2393.

[30] Bhat S. A., Mague J. T., Balakrishna M. S., Transition metal chemistry of large-bite bisphosphines, *N,N*-bis(diphenylphosphinobenzyl)-*N*-phenylamine and bis(2-diphenylphosphinobenzyl)ether, *J. Organomet. Chem.*, 2016, 809, 21-30.

[31] Sarcher C., Bestgen S., Falk F. C., Lebedkin S., Pradies J., Roesky P. W., Synthesis and photophysical properties of GemPhos noble metal complexes, *J. Organomet. Chem.,* 2015, 795, 11-17.

[32] Zubiri M. R., Milton H. L., Cole-Hamilton D. J., Slawin A. M. Z., Woollins J. D., The preparation and complexation of 5,10-

bis(diphenylphosphino)phenazine, *Inorg. Chem. Commun.*, 2004, 7, 201-203.

[33] Melník M., Holloway C. E., Stereochemistry of platinum(II) coordination compounds, *Coord. Chem. Rev.*, 2006, 250, 2261-2270.

In: New Developments in Oncology Research ISBN: 978-1-53615-365-1
Editor: Marcos T. Blair © 2019 Nova Science Publishers, Inc.

Chapter 4

ORGANODIPHOSPHINES IN CIS-PT(η^2-PXP)(CL)$_2$ AND CIS-PT(η^2-PXXP)(CL)$_2$ DERIVATIVES: STRUCTURAL ASPECTS

Milan Melník, Andrea Forgácsová and Peter Mikuš
Department of Pharmaceutical Analysis and Nuclear Pharmacy, Faculty of Pharmacy, Comenius University in Bratislava, Bratislava, Slovak Republic
Toxicological and Antidoping Center, Faculty of Pharmacy, Comenius University in Bratislava, Bratislava, Slovak Republic

ABSTRACT

This chapter covers eighty five Pt(II) complexes with an inner coordination sphere of cis-PtP_2Cl_2. The P-donor ligands are organodiphosphines which create four- and five-membered metallocyclic rings with the PCP, PNP, PC-CP, PC=CP, PN_2P and PCOP types. The effects of both steric and electronic factors can be seen from the values of the P-Pt-P bite angles, with the mean values: 74.4° (PCP), 71.8° (PNP), 87.3° (PC-CP), 86.5° (PC=CP), 84.3° (PN_2P) and 84.0° (PCOP). The mean value of Pt-P bond distance of 2.217 Å (trans to Cl) is much shorter (more covalent) than the mean value of Pt-Cl bond distance of 2.364 Å (trans to P), as a reason of stronger trans- influence of P over Cl. There are complexes which are examples of distortion and ligand isomerism.

Keywords: structures, cis-PtP_2Cl_2, organodiphosphines, isomers, review

ABBREVIATIONS

$(C_5H_{10}N)_2P(C_5H_8)P(C_5H_{10}N)_2$	1,2-bis(bis(piperidin-1-yl) phosphino)cyclopentane
$(C_6H_2Bu^t_3)P(C_{16}H_{10})P(C_6H_2Bu^t_3)$	(3,4-diphenylcyclobut-3-ene-1,3-diylidene)bis(2,4,6-tri-t-butylphenyl)phosphine
$(C_6H_4NMe_2\text{-}2)_2P(CH_2)_2P(C_6H_4NMe_2\text{-}2)_2$	1,2-bis(bis(bis(/2-dimethylamino) phenyl) phosphine)
$(C_6H_5NO)_2PN(Me)N(Me)P(C_6H_5NO)_2{}^*$	(bis(bis(6-methylpyridin-2-yl)oxy) phosphino)-1,2-dimethylhydrazine
$(\eta^2\text{-}C_6H_{12})P(CH_2)_2P(\eta^2\text{-}C_6H_{12})$	1,1'-ethane-1,2-diylbis(3,5-dimethylphospholane)
$(C_7H_7O)_2PN(Me)N(Me)P(C_7H_7O)_2$	bis(1,2-bis(bis(2-methoxyphenyl phosphino)-1,2-dimethylhydrazine)
$(C_7H_9N_2)P_2(C_6H_4)P(C_7H_9N_2)_2$	(N,N′,N",N‴-(1,2-phenylene-bis(phosphinetriyl-P) bis(methylene))-tetrakis(N-methylpyridin-2-amine)
$C_{16}H_{16}P_2$	1,1′-diphenyl-3,3′,4,4′-tetramethyl-2,2′-biphosphole
$(\eta^2\text{-}C_{20}H_{12}O_2)PN(Me)N(Me)P(\eta^2\text{-}C_{20}H_{12}O_2$	N,N′-bis(dinaphtho(2,1-d:1′,2′-f)(1,3,2)dioxa phosphepin-2-yl)-1,2-dimethylhydrazine
$(\eta^2\text{-}C_{28}H_{16}O_2)O(CH_2)_2O(\eta^2\text{-}C_{28}H_{16}O_2)$	1,2-bis(9,9′-biphenanthrolyl phosphonito)ethane
$(Me)(Bu^t)P(C_8H_4N_2)P(Bu^t)(Me)$	2,3-bis(t-butyl(methyl)phosphino) quinoxaline

(Ph)(Cl)P($C_2H_1B_{10}$)P(Cl)(Ph)	1,2-bis(chloro(phenyl)phosphino)-1,2-dicarba-closo-dodecarborane
$(PhO)_2$/N(Me)N(Me)P$(OPh)_2$	bis(1,2-bis(diphenylphosphito)-1,2-dimethylhydrazine
$(PhO)_2$P(C_5H_8)PPh_2	1,2-bis(bis(phenoxy)phosphino) cyclopentane
Ph_2CH(CN)PPh_2	bis(diphenylphosphino)acetonitrile
Ph_2P($C_{10}H_{11}O$)PPh	6-(diphenylphosphino)-8,9-dimethyl-10-phenyl-3-oxa-10-phosphatricyclo [5.2.1.0^{2,5}]deca-4,8-diene
Ph_2P($C_{10}H_{13}O_2$)PPh	6-(diphenylphosphino)-8,9-dimethyl-10-phenyl-3-oxa-10-phosphatricyclo [5.2.1.0^{2,6}]dec-8-en-4-ol
Ph_2P($C_{10}H_{15}O$)PPh	5,6-dimethyl-7-phenyl-2-(diphenylphosphino)-7-phosphabicyclo(2.2.1) hept-5-en-2-yl)ethanol
Ph_2P($C_{20}H_{10}O_3$)PPh_2	2-((9-anthracenyl)methylene)-4,5-bis(diphenyl-phosphino)-4-cyclopenten-1,3-dione
Ph_2P($C_{22}H_{10}O_2$)PPh_2	4,5-bis(diphenylphosphino)-2-(pyren-1-ylmethylene) cyclopent-4-ene-1,3-dione
Ph_2P($C_3H_3N_3$)PEt_2	4-(diisopropylphosphino)-5-diphenylphosphino)-2-methyl-2H-1,2,3-triazole
Ph_2P($C_4H_8Ph_2$)PPh_2	1,2-bis(diphenylphosphanyl)-3,4-diphenylcyclobutane
Ph_2P($C_5H_2O_2$)PPh_2	4,5-bis(diphenylphosphino)-4-cyclopenten-1,3-diene
Ph_2P(C_6H_4)P(η^2-C_6H_{12})	1-(2,5-dimethylphospholano)-2-(diphenylphosphino)-1,2-phenylene

$Ph_2P(C_6H_6O)P(CH{=}CH_2)(Ph)$	4-(diphenyphosphino)-5-((ethenyl(phenyl)phosphino)-7-oxabicyclo[2.2.1]hept-2-ene
$Ph_2P(C_6H_8O)PPh_2$	4,5-bis(diphenylphosphino)-7-oxbicyclo[2.2.1]heptane
$Ph_2P(C_9H_{13}O)PPh$	5,6-dimethyl-7-phenyl-2-(diphenylphosphino)-phosphabicyclo (2.2.1)hept-5-en-2-yl)methanol
$Ph_2P(C_9H_6)PBu^t_2$	(di-t-butyl(3-diphenylphosphino)-1H-inden-2-yl)phosphine)
$Ph_2P(CH_2)_2P(\eta^2\text{-}C_6H_{12})$	(1-(2´,5´-dimethylphospholano-2-(diphenylphosphino) ethane
$Ph_2P\{C(COOMe){=}C(COOMe)\}PBu^t_2$	1-(di-t-butylphosphino)-2-(diphenyl-phosphino)-1,2-bis(methoxycarbonyl)ethene
$Ph_2P\{CH{=}C(COOEt)\}P(\eta^2\text{-}C_{18}H_{20}N_2)$	2-(1,3-bis(2,6-dimethylphenyl)-2,3-dihydro-1H-1,3,2-diazaphospho-2-yl)-3-(diphenylphosphino)acrylic acid etyl ester
$Ph_2PCH(Me)CH(Me)PPh_2$	bis(diphenylphosphino)butane
$Ph_2PCH(Me)P(OH)(2,4,6\text{-}Bu^t_3C_6H_3)$	1-hydroxy-2-methyl-2,3-diphenyl-1-(1,4,6-tri-t-butylphenyl)-1,3-diphosphapropane
$Ph_2PN(C_{10}H_7)PPh_2$	N-(diphenylphosphino)-N-1-naphthyl-P,P-dipheny-lphosphinous amide
$Ph_2PN(C_6H_4CN\text{-}2)PPh_2$	2-cyanophenyliminotetraphenyl diphosphane
$Ph_2PN(C_6H_4COOMe\text{-}3)PPh_2$	(3-methoxycarbonylphenyl)bis (diphenylphosphino)amine
$Ph_2PN(C_6H_4Et\text{-}2)PPh_2$	N,N-bis(diphenylphosphino-2-ethylaniline
$Ph_2PN(C_6H_4Ph\text{-}2)PPh_2$	N,N-bis(diphenylphosphino-2-phenylaniline

$Ph_2PN(CH_2C_4H_3O)PPh_2$	N-(diphenylphosphino)-N-(2-furylmethyl)P,Pdiphenyl-phosphinous amide
$Ph_2PN(CH_2C_5H_4N)PPh_2$	2-(bis(diphenylphosphino) aminomethyl)pyridine
$Ph_2PN(CH_2CH{=}CH_2)PPh_2$	bis(diphenylphosphino) (2-propenyl)amine)
$Ph_2PN(CH_2Et)PPh_2$	N,N-bis(diphenylphosphino) propylamine
$Ph_2PN(CH_2Ph)PPh_2$	(benzylbis)(diphenylphosphino)amine
$Ph_2PN\{(CH_2)_2SCH_2Ph\}PPh_2$	((2-benzylthio)ethyl)bis (diphenylphosphino)amine
$Ph_2PN\{C_6H_3(Me)_2\text{-}2,3\}PPh_2$	N,N-bis(diphenylphosphino)-2,3-dimethylaniline
$Ph_2PN\{CH(Me)(COOMe)\}PPh_2$	N,N-bi(diphenylphosphino)alanine methylester
$Ph_2PN\{CH(Me)(Et)\}PPh_2$	N,N-bis(diphenylphosphanyl)-sec-butylamine
$PhP(CH_2)(CH_2Si(CH_3)_2CH_2)PPh$	5,5-dimethyl-1,3-diphenyl-1,3,5-diphosphasilinan-1,3-diyl
$Pr^i_2O(C_2H_{10}B_{10})PPr^i_2$	1,2-bis(diisopropylphosphino-1,2-dicarba-closo-dodecaborane
$Pr^i_2P(o\text{-}C_6H_4)PPr^i_2$	bis(diisopropylphosphino)o-phenylene
$Pr^i_2P(OCH_2)P(\eta^2\text{-}C_{10}H_{16}O_3)$	((1,3,5,7-tetramethyl-2,4,6-trioxa-8-phosphatricyclo [3.3.1.1^{3,7}]dec-8-yl)methyl)di-isopropylphosphinite
$(2\text{-}Pr^i_2C_6H_4)_2P(CH_2)P(2\text{-}Pr^i_2C_6H_4)_2$	(bis(bis(2-isopropylphenyl) phosphino)methane

1. Introduction

The chemistry of platinum is an important area particularly in the fields of biochemistry, catalysis and theory. The chemistry of platinum coordination complexes has been extensively investigated over the last haft century, especially the relationship between the structure and reactivity. The over helming majority of X-ray structural studies of square planar transition metal complexes are of platinum complexes. Although the most common oxidation state of platinum is +2, the metal is also found in 0, +1, +3, +4, +5 and non- integral oxidation states. Over two thousand and five hundred platinum complexes have been reviewed [1]. About 10% of these complexes exist as isomers and were summarized and analyzed [2]. Included are distortion (65%), cis- trans (30%), mixed isomers and ligand isomerism.

Organophosphines are very attractive and useful ligands forming wide variability of stereochemistry about central transition metals and platinum is no exception. Recently we analyzed structural parameters of organomonophosphines in monomeric PtP_2Cl_2 derivatives [3]. In this review we classify and analyze structural parameters of monomeric PtP_2Cl_2 complexes in which P-donor ligands are organodiphosphines. Therefore that organodiphosphines form wide variability of n-membered metallocycles in this review is analyze only such organodisphosphines which form four- and five-membered metallocycles. The primary source of information was Cambridge Crystallographic Database up to the end of 2017.

2. Cis-PtP_2Cl_2 Derivatives

There are over eighty five monomeric Pt(II) complexes with such chromophore for which structural parameters are available. In these derivatives a square planar environment about each Pt(II) atom is build up by homobidentate-P,P' donor ligands together with a pair of chlorine atoms with varying degrees of distortion.

2.1. Pt(η^2-PXP)(Cl)$_2$ Type

There are two types of the chelating-P,P' donor ligands which form four-membered metallocycles: PCP and PNP.

2.1.1. Pt(η^2-PCP)(Cl)$_2$ Type

There are five complexes, mostly colorless which crystallized in two crystal systems: orthorhombic (x1) and monoclinic (x4), contain organodiphosphine ligands which form four- membered (PCP) metallocyclic rings. Such complexes are: [Pt{η^2-$Bu^t_2PCH_2PBu^t_2$}$(Cl)_2$] [4], [Pt{η^2-$Ph_2PCH_2PPh_2$}$(Cl)_2$] [5], [Pt{η^2-$Ph_2PCH(CN)PPh_2$}$(Cl)_2$].$2CH_2Cl_2$ [6], [Pt{η^2-(2-$Pr^i_2C_6H_4)_2PCH_2P$(2-$Pr^i_2C_6H_4)_2$}$(Cl)_2$].CH_2Cl_2 [7] and [Pt{η^2-$Ph_2PCH(Me)P(OH)$.(2,4,6-$Bu^t_3C_6H_3$)}$(Cl)_2$].EtOH.C_4H_8O [8]. Structure of [Pt{η^2-$Ph_2PCH(CN)PPh_2$}$(Cl)_2$] [6] is shown in Figure 1 as an example. The mean value of P-Pt-P bite angles is 74.4° (PCP). The mean values of the remaining L-Pt-L bond angles are 90.3° (Cl-Pt-Cl), 96.6° and 173.2° (P-Pt-Cl). The mean values of Pt-L bond distances are 2.230 Å (P, trans to Cl) and 2.355 Å (Cl, trans to P).

2.1.2. Pt(η^2-PNP)(Cl)$_2$ Type

There are nineteen complexes, mostly pale yellow, which crystallized in three crystal systems: triclinic (x1), orthorhombic (x4) and monoclinic (x14), and contain chelating-P,P donor ligands build up four-membered (PNP) metallocycles. Such complexes are: [Pt{(η^2-$Ph_2PN(Me)PPh_2$}$(Cl)_2$] [9], [Pt{(η^2-$Ph_2PN(CH_2Et)PPh_2$}$(Cl)_2$] [10], [Pt{(η^2-$Ph_2PN(CH_2CH{=}CH_2)$ PPh_2}$(Cl)_2$] [11], [Pt{(η^2-$Ph_2PN(CH_2Ph)PPh_2$}$(Cl)_2$].CH_2Cl_2 [12], [Pt{(η^2-$Ph_2PN(CH_2C_5H_4N)PPh_2$}$(Cl)_2$].CH_2Cl_2 [12], [Pt{(η^2-Ph_2PN{$(CH_2)_2$ SCH_2Ph} PPh_2}$(Cl)_2$] [13], [Pt{(η^2-Ph_2PN{CH(Me)(COOMe)}PPh_2}$(Cl)_2$] [14], [Pt{(η^2-Ph_2PN{CH(Me)(Et)}PPh_2}$(Cl)_2$] [15], [Pt{(η^2-Ph_2PN (C_6H_4CN-2)PPh_2}$(Cl)_2$] [16], [Pt{(η^2-$Ph_2PN(C_6H_4CN$-3)PPh_2}$(Cl)_2$]. CH_2Cl_2 [17], [Pt{(η^2-$Ph_2PN(C_6H_4CN$-4)PPh_2}$(Cl)_2$].CH_2Cl_2 [17], [Pt{(η^2-$Ph_2PN(C_6H_4Ph$-2)PPh_2}$(Cl)_2$].$CHCl_3$ [17], [Pt{(η^2-$Ph_2PN(C_6H_4Et$-3)PPh_2} $(Cl)_2$].$CHCl_3$ [18], [Pt{(η^2-$Ph_2PN(C_6H_4Pr^i$-2)PPh_2}$(Cl)_2$].Et_2O [19], [Pt{(η^2-$Ph_2PN(C_6H_4COOMe$-3)PPh_2}$(Cl)_2$].$CHCl_3$ [20], [Pt{(η^2-Ph_2PN{$C_6H_3(Me)_2$-2,3}PPh_2}$(Cl)_2$].$CHCl_3$ [21], [Pt{(η^2-Ph_2PN{$C_6H_3(Me)_2$-2,5}PPh_2}$(Cl)_2$] [21], [Pt{(η^2-$Ph_2PN(CH_2C_4H_3O)PPh_2$}$(Cl)_2$].CH_2Cl_2 [22], and [Pt{(η^2-$Ph_2PN(C_{10}H_7)PPh_2$}$(Cl)_2$].Me_2CO [23]. Structure of [Pt{(η^2-Ph_2PN $(CH_2Ph)PPh_2$}$(Cl)_2$] [12] is shown in Figure 2 as an example. The mean value of P-Pt-P bite angles is 71.8° (PNP). The mean values of the remaining

L-Pt-L bond angles are 92.2° (Cl-Pt-Cl), 97.5° and 169.7° (P-Pt-Cl). The mean values of Pt-L bond distances are 2.210 Å (P, trans to Cl) and 2.354 Å (Cl, trans to P).

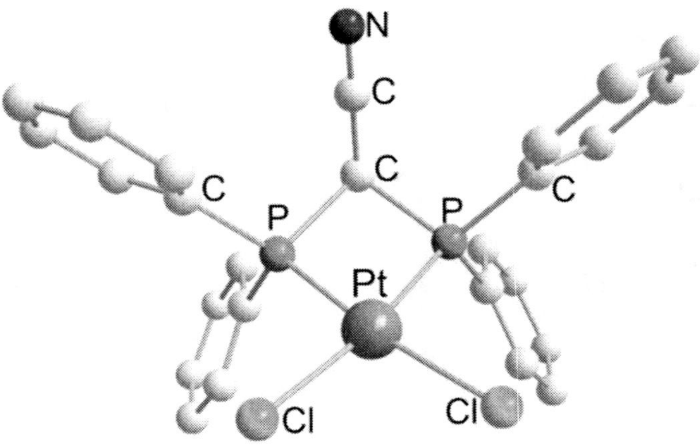

Figure 1. Structure of [Pt{η^2-$Ph_2PCH(CN)PPh_2$}$(Cl)_2$] [6].

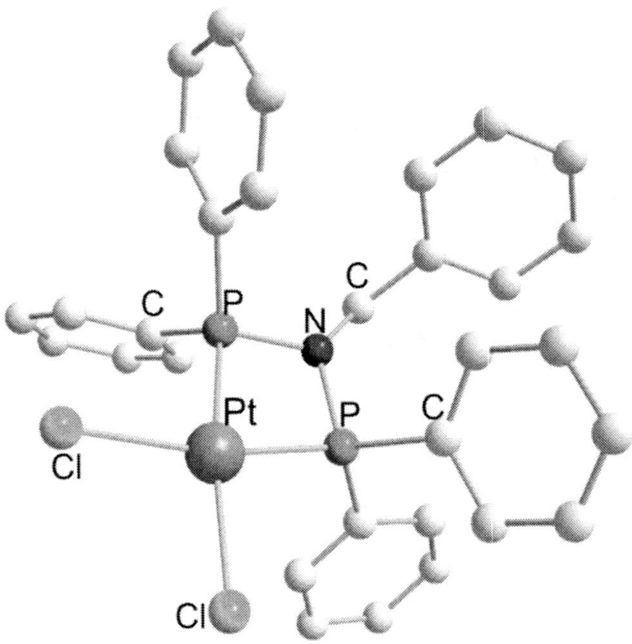

Figure 2. Structure of [Pt{(η^2-$Ph_2PN(CH_2Ph)PPh_2$}$(Cl)_2$] [12].

2.2. Pt(η^2-PXXP)(Cl)$_2$ Type

Organodiphosphine ligands which build up five-membered metallocyclic rings can be divided into the four types: PC-CP (saturated), PC=CP (unsaturated), PNNP and POCP and together with a pair of chlorine atoms form a distorted square planar environment about each Pt(II) atom (cis-PtP_2Cl_2). These complexes crystallized in four crystal systems: tetragonal (x2), triclinic (x10), orthorhombic (x16) and monoclinic (x33).

2.2.1. Pt(η^2-PC-CP)(Cl)$_2$ Type

There are thirty three examples in which organodiphosphine ligands build up saturated five-membered metallocyclic rings (PC-CP): [Pt{η^2-$Et_2P(CH_2)_2PEt_2$}(Cl)$_2$] [24], [Pt{η^2-$Bu^t{}_2P(CH_2)_2PBu^t{}_2$}(Cl)$_2$] (monoclinic, at 100K) [25], and (monoclinic at 298K) [26], [Pt{η^2-$Bu^t{}_2P(CH_2)_2PBu^t{}_2$} (Cl)$_2$]PhCl [26], [Pt{$\eta^2$-$Ph_2P(CH_2)_2PPh_2$}(Cl)$_2$ (monoclinic [27], [Pt{η^2-$Ph_2P(CH_2)_2PPh_2$}(Cl)$_2$].CH_2Cl_2 [28], [Pt{η^2-$Ph_2P(CH_2)_2PPh_2$}(Cl)$_2$] (monoclinic) [29], [Pt{η^2-$Ph_2P(CH_2)_2PPh_2$}(Cl)$_2$] (monoclinic) [30], [Pt{η^2-$Ph_2P(CH_2)_2PPh_2$}(Cl)$_2$] (orthorhombic, at 150K) [31], [Pt{η^2-$cy_2P(CH_2)_2Pcy_2$}(Cl)$_2$] [32], [Pt{η^2-(Ph)(OH)P$(CH_2)_2$P(OH)(Ph)}(Cl)$_2$] [33], [Pt{η^2-$(C_6H_4NMe_2$-2)$_2$P$(CH_2)_2$P($C_6H_4NMe_2$-2}(Cl)$_2$].CH_2Cl_2 [34], [Pt{η^2-($C_6H_4Pr^i$-2)$_2$P$(CH_2)_2$P($C_6H_4Pr^i$-2)$_2$}(Cl)$_2$].CH_2Cl_2 [35], [Pt{η^2-$Ph_2P(CH_2)_2P(\eta^2$-$C_6H_{12})$}(Cl)$_2$] [36], [Pt{η^2-(η^2-C_6H_{12})P$(CH_2)_2$P(η^2-C_6H_{12})} (Cl)$_2$] [37], [Pt{η^2-(η^2-$C_{28}H_{16}O_2$)P$(CH_2)_2$P(η^2-$C_{28}H_{16}O_2$)}(Cl)$_2$]. CH_2Cl_2 [38], [Pt{η^2-Ph_2PCH(Me)CH(Me)PPh_2}(Cl)$_2$] [39], [Pt{η^2-$Ph_2P(C_4H_4Ph_2)$ PPh_2}(Cl)$_2$] [40], [Pt{η^2-$(PhO)_2P(C_5H_8)(OPh)_2$}(Cl)$_2$] (monoclinic) [41], [Pt{η^2-$(PhO)_2P(C_5H_8)(OPh)_2$}(Cl)$_2$] (monoclinic) [41], [Pt{η^2-$(C_5H_{10}N)$ $_2P(C_5H_8)P(C_5H_{10}N)_2$}(Cl)$_2$] [41], [Pt{$\eta^2$-$Ph_2P(\eta^3$-$C_9H_{13}O)$ PPh}(Cl)$_2$]. CH_2Cl_2 [42], [Pt{η^2-$Ph_2P(\eta^3$-$C_{10}H_{15}O)$PPh}(Cl)$_2$] [42], [Pt{η^2-$Ph_2P(\eta^3$-$C_{10}H_{11}O)$PPh}(Cl)$_2$] [43], [Pt{η^2-$Ph_2P(\eta^3$-$C_{10}H_{13}O)$PPh}(Cl)$_2$]. $CHCl_3$ [43], [Pt{η^2-$Ph_2P(C_6H_8O)PPh_2$}(Cl)$_2$] [44], [Pt{η^2-$Ph_2P(C_6H_8O)$ PEt_2}(Cl)$_2$] [45], [Pt{η^2-$Ph_2P(C_6H_6O)P(CH{=}CH_2)(Ph)$}(Cl)$_2$] [45], [Pt{$\eta^2$-$Ph_2P(C_3H_3N_3)$ PEt_2}(Cl)$_2$] [46], [Pt{η^2-$Pr^i{}_2P(C_2H_{10}B_{10})PPr^i{}_2$}(Cl)$_2$].$CH_2Cl_2$ [47], [Pt{η^2-(Ph)(Cl)P$(C_2H_{10}B_{10})$P(Cl)(Ph)}(Cl)$_2$].toluene [48], [Pt{η^2-(Et_2N)(Cl)P

$(C_2H_{10}B_{10})P(Cl)(NEt_2)\}(Cl)_2]$.toluene [48], and $[Pt\{\eta^2\text{-}(Bu^t)(Cl)P\ (C_2H_{10}B_{10})P(Cl)(Bu^t)\}(Cl)_2]$ [48]. Structure of $[Pt\{\eta^2\text{-}Ph_2P(CH_2)_2P(\eta^2\text{-}C_6H_{12})\}(Cl)_2]$ [36] is shown in Figure 3 as an example. The mean value of P-Pt-P bite angles is 87.3° (PC-CP). The mean values of the remaining L-Pt-L bond angles are 82.2° (Cl-Pt-Cl), 92.5° and 176.6° (P-Pt-Cl). The mean values of Pt-L bond distances are: 2.225 Å (P, trans to Cl) and 2.362 Å (Cl, trans to P).

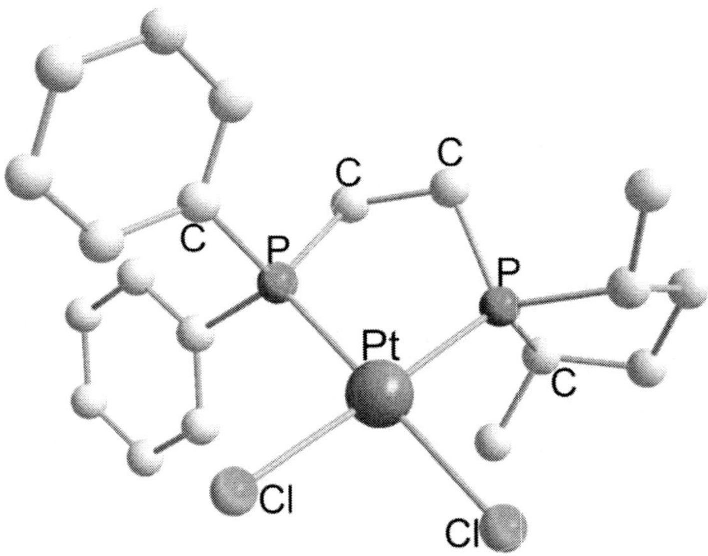

Figure 3. Structure of $[Pt\{\eta^2\text{-}Ph_2P(CH_2)_2P(\eta^2\text{-}C_6H_{12})\}(Cl)_2]$ [36].

2.2.2. *Cis- $Pt(\eta^2\text{-}PC{=}CP)(Cl)_2$ Type*

There are fifteen examples in which organodiphosphine ligands create unsaturated five-membered metallocyclic rings (PC=CP). Such complexes are: $[Pt\{\eta^2\text{-}Ph_2P\{C(COOMe){=}C(COOMe)\}PBu^t_2\}(Cl)_2].CHCl_3$ [49], $[Pt\{\eta^2\text{-}Ph_2P\{C(COOMe){=}C(COOMe)\}Pcy_2\}(Cl)_2].CH_2Cl_2$ [49], $[Pt\{\eta^2\text{-}cy_2P\{C(COOMe){=}C(COOMe)\}Pcy_2\}(Cl)_2].CHCl_3$ [49], $[Pt\{\eta^2\text{-}Ph_2P(C_9H_3)PBu^t_2\}(Cl)_2]$ [50], $[Pt\{\eta^2\text{-}Pr^i_2P(C_6H_4)PPr^i_2\}(Cl)_2]$ [51], $[Pt\{\eta^2\text{-}(C_7H_9N_2)_2P(C_6H_4)P(C_7H_9N_2)_2\}(Cl)_2]$ [52], $[Pt\{\eta^2\text{-}Ph_2P(C_6H_4)P(\eta^2\text{-}C_6H_{12})\}(Cl)_2].CH_2Cl_2$ [53], $[Pt\{\eta^2\text{-}(Bu^t)(Me)P(C_8H_4N_2)P(Me)(Bu^t)\}(Cl)_2].CH_2Cl_2$ [54], $[Pt\{\eta^2\text{-}Ph_2P(C_5H_2O_2)PPh_2\}(Cl)_2]$ [55], $[Pt\{\eta^2\text{-}Ph_2P(C_{20}H_{10}O_2)PPh_2\}(Cl)_2]$.

CH_2Cl_2 [55], [Pt{η^2-$Ph_2P(C_{22}H_{10}O_2)PPh_2$}$(Cl)_2$].$CH_2Cl_2$ [56], [Pt{η^2-Ph_2P{CH=C(COOEt)P(η^2-$C_{18}H_{20}N_2$)}$(Cl)_2$].C_6H_6 [57], [Pt{η^2-$C_{16}H_{16}P_2$}$(Cl)_2$] [58], [Pt{η^2-methyldiphos}$(Cl)_2$] [59], and [Pt{η^2-($C_6H_2Bu^t{}_3$)P($C_{16}H_{10}$)P($C_6H_2Bu^t{}_3$)}$(Cl)_2$].Me_2CO [60]. Structure of [Pt{η^2-cy_2P{C(COOMe)=C(COOMe)}Pcy_2}$(Cl)_2$] [49] is shown in Figure 4 as an example. The mean value of P-Pt-P bite angles is 86.5° (PC=CP). The mean values of the remaining L-Pt-L bond angles are 91.5° (Cl-PtCl), 90.8° and 175.8° (P-Pt-Cl). The mean values of Pt-L bond distances are 2.221 Å (P, trans to Cl) and 2.354 Å (Cl, trans to P).

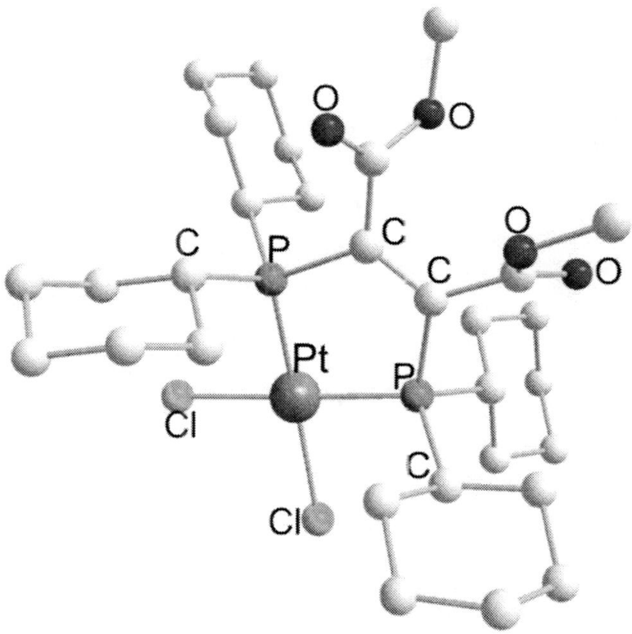

Figure 4. Structure of [Pt{η^2-cy_2P{C(COOMe)=C(COOMe)}Pcy_2}$(Cl)_2$] [49].

2.2.3. *Cis- Pt(η^2-PNNP)(Cl)$_2$ Type*

There are eleven examples mostly yellow, in which organodiphosphine donor ligands form five-membered metallocyclic rings of the (PNNP) type and together with a pair of chlorine atoms completed a distorted square planar environment about each Pt(II) atom. Such complexes are: [Pt{η^2-$(PhO)_2$PN(Me)N(Me)P$(OPh)_2$}$(Cl)_2$] [61], [Pt{η^2-(η^2-$C_{12}H_{10}$)PN(Me)

N(Me)P(η^2-$C_{12}H_{10}$)}(Cl)$_2$] [61], [Pt{η^2-(C_6H_5NO)$_2$PN(Me)N(Me)P(C_6H_5NO)$_2$}(Cl)$_2$] (orthorhombic and triclinic) [62], [Pt{η^2-(Cl)$_2$PN(Me)N(Me)P(Cl)$_2$}(Cl)$_2$] [63], [Pt{η^2-(η^2-$C_{20}H_{12}O_2$)PN(Me)N(Me)P(η^2-$C_{20}H_{12}O_2$)}(Cl)$_2$].2H_2O [64], [Pt{η^2-(PhO)$_2$PN(Et)N(Et)P(OPh)$_2$}(Cl)$_2$] [65], [Pt{η^2-(C_7H_7O)$_2$PN(Me)N(Me)P(C_7H_7O)$_2$}(Cl)$_2$].CH_2Cl_2 [65], [Pt{η^2-(C_7H_7O)$_2$PN(Et)N(Et)P(C_7H_7O)$_2$}(Cl)$_2$].CH_2Cl_2.H_2O [65], and [Pt{η^2-Ph$_2$PN(Ph)N(Ph)PPh$_2$}(Cl)$_2$].$CHCl_3$ [66]. Structure of [Pt{η^2-Ph$_2$PN(Ph)N(Ph)PPh$_2$}(Cl)$_2$] [66] is shown in Figure 5 as an example. The mean value of P-Pt-P bite angles is 84.3° (PNNP). The mean values of the remaining L-Pt-L bond angles are 90.5° (Cl-Pt-Cl), 92.5° and 176.0° (P-Pt-Cl). The mean values of Pt-L bond distances are 2.194 Å (P, trans to Cl) and 2.344 Å (Cl, trans to P).

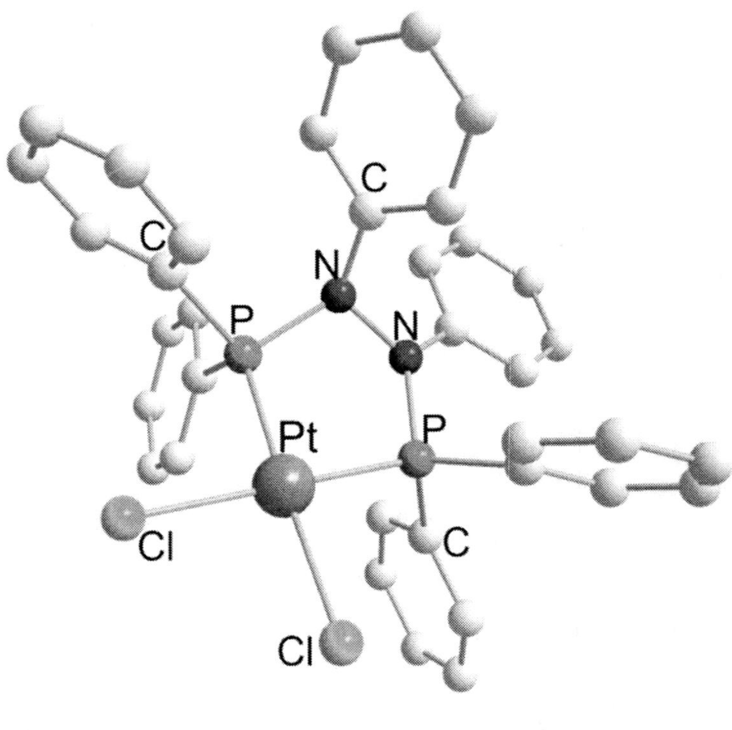

Figure 5. Structure of [Pt{η^2-Ph$_2$PN(Ph)N(Ph)PPh$_2$}(Cl)$_2$] [66].

2.2.4. Cis- Pt(η^2-PCOP)(Cl)$_2$ Type

There are two triclinic examples: [Pt{η^2-Pr$^i_2$P(OCH$_2$)P(η^2-C$_{10}$H$_{16}$O$_3$)}(Cl)$_2$] [67] and [Pt{η^2-Ph$_2$P(OCH$_2$)P(η^2-C$_{10}$H$_{16}$O$_3$)}(Cl)$_2$]. CHCl$_3$ [67] in which organodiphosphine donor ligands form five-membered metallocyclic rings of PCOP type. Structure of [Pt{η^2-Pr$^i_2$P(OCH$_2$)P(η^2-C$_{10}$H$_{16}$O$_3$)}(Cl)$_2$] [67] is shown in Figure 6 as an example. The mean value of P-Pt-P bite angle is 84.0° (PCOP). The mean values of Pt-L bond distances are 2.22 Å (P, trans to Cl) and 2.355 Å (Cl, trans to P). The mean values of remaining L-Pt-L bond angles are 94.0° (Cl-Pt-Cl), 95.2° and 175.0° (P-Pt-Cl).

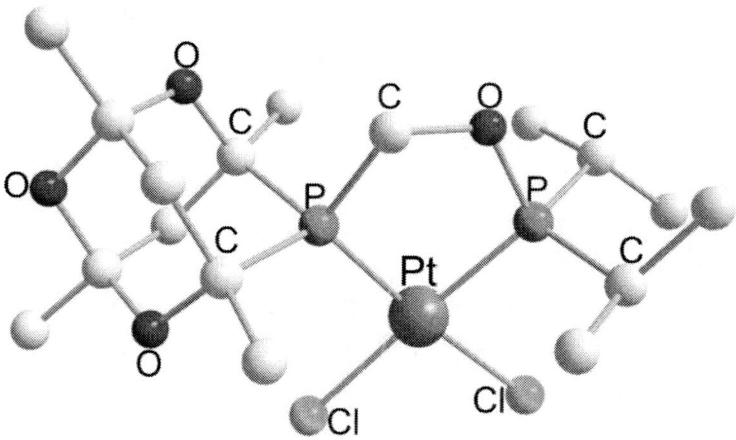

Figure 6. Structure of [Pt{η^2-Pr$^i_2$P(OCH$_2$)P(η^2-C$_{10}$H$_{16}$O$_3$)}(Cl)$_2$] [67].

CONCLUSION

This review includes eighty five coordination compounds of platinum, in which each Pt(II) atom is in a distorted square planar environment with inner coordination sphere of cis-PtP$_2$Cl$_2$. These complexes crystallized in four crystal systems: tetragonal (x2), triclinic (x13), orthorhombic (x20) and monoclinic (x50). The P-donor ligands are organobiphosphines which create four- and five-membered metallocycles. The former create two types metallocycles: PCP and PNP, the latter create four types of metallocycles PC-CP, PC=CP, PN_2P and PCOP. The mean values of L-Pt-L bite angles are: 74.4° (PCP), 71.8° (PNP), 87.3° (PC-CP), 86.5° (PC=CP), 84.3° (PN_2P) and 84.0° (PCOP).

The mean value of Pt-P bond distance of 2.217 Å (P, trans to Cl) is more stronger (covalent) than the Pt-Cl bond distance of 2.364 Å (Cl, trans to P) as a reason of much stronger trans-influence of P over Cl atom.

Two types of isomerism exist in these derivatives. There are examples: $[Pt\{\eta^2\text{-}Ph_2PN(C_6H_4CN\text{-}2)PPh_2\}(Cl)_2]$ [16], $[Pt\{\eta^2\text{-}Ph_2PN(C_6H_4CN\text{-}3)PPh_2\}(Cl)_2]$ [17], $[Pt\{\eta^2\text{-}Ph_2PN(C_6H_4CN\text{-}4)PPh_2\}(Cl)_2]$ [17], and $[Pt\{\eta^2\text{-}Ph_2PN\{C_6H_3(Me)_2\text{-}2,3\}PPh_2\}(Cl)_2]$ [21], $[Pt\{\eta^2\text{-}Ph_2PN\{C_6H_3(Me)_2\text{-}2,5\}PPh_2\}(Cl)_2]$ [21]; and $[Pt\{\eta^2\text{-}(C_6H_5NO)_2PN(Me)N(Me)P(C_6H_5NO)_2\}(Cl)_2]$ [61], $[Pt\{\eta^2\text{-}(C_6H_5NO)_2PN(Me)N(Me)P(C_6H_5NO_2^*)_2\ (Cl)_2]$ [61], which are classical examples of ligand isomerism.

Another several complexes: $[Pt\{\eta^2\text{-}Bu^t_2P(CH_2)_2PBu^t_2\}(Cl)_2]$ (monoclinic) at 100K [25] and at 298K [26]; $[Pt\{\eta^2\text{-}Ph_2P(CH_2)_2PPh_2\}(Cl)_2]$ (monoclinic) at 298K [29,30] and (orthorhombic) at 150K [31]; $[Pt\{\eta^2\text{-}(PhO)_2P(C_5H_8)P(OPh)_2\}(Cl)_2]$ (two monoclinic) [41]; and $[Pt\{\eta^2\text{-}(C_6H_5NO)_2PN(Me)N(Me)P(C_6H_5NO)_2\}(Cl)_2]$ orthorhombic and monoclinic [62] which are classical examples of distortion isomerism [2].

There is cooperative effect between the structural parameters of the complexes with four- and five-membered metallocyclic rings. When P-Pt-P bite angle opens the cis-Cl-Pt-Cl and cis-P-Pt-Cl bond angles closes with the total mean values which opening in the orders: 72.4° (PXP) < 91.7° (Cl-Pt-Cl) < 97.3° (P-Pt-Cl) vs 86.9° (PX_2P) < 88.0° (Cl-Pt-Cl) < 92.7° (P-Pt-Cl). In general complexes with four-membered metallocycles are more distorted than with five-membered metallocycles, as expected.

During the collection and organization of the data it has become evident that in spite of the increasing availability of data retrieval systems, the tracking of relevant structural data is not always simple. Poorly chosen key words for indexes appear to be one problem which results in effective invisibility of some material from a structural point of view. Some original papers are lacking important information such as atomic coordinates and analysis of intermolecular distances. Increasingly such data are also being relegated to supplementary material. In view of those limitations we believe that such review such as this can continue to serve useful function by centralizing available material and delimiting areas worthy of further investigation.

Acknowledgments

This work was supported by the projects VEGA 1/0873/15, KEGA 022UK-4/2015, APVV-15-0585.

References

[1] Holloway C. E., Melník M., Structural Aspect of Platinum Coordination Compounds: Part I. Monomeric Pt°, Pt1 and PtnA4 Derivatives. *Rev. Inorg. Chem.,* 2002, *22*, pp 163-284.; Structural Aspect of Platinum Coordination Compounds: Part II. Monomeric Pt11 Compounds with PtA3B and PtA2B2 Composition. *Rev. Inorg. Chem.,* 2003, *23*, pp 125-287; Structural aspect of platinum coordination compounds: Part III. Monomeric square planar (PtA2XY and PtABXY) and trigonal bipyramidal PtII coordination compounds. *Rev. Inorg. Chem.,* 2004, *24*, pp 135-299; Structural aspect of platinum coordination compounds: Part IV. Monomeric square PtIII and PtIV coordination compounds. *Rev. Inorg. Chem.,* 2004, *24*, pp 301-400; Structural aspect of platinum coordination compounds: Part V. Dimeric and oligomeric platinum derivatives. *Rev. Inorg. Chem.,* 2005, *25*, pp 93-270.

[2] Melník M., Holloway C. E., Stereochemistry of platinum coordination compounds. *Coord. Chem. Rev.*, 2006, *250*, pp 2261-2270.

[3] Melník M., Mikuš P., Organomonophosphines in PtP2Cl2 derivatives: structural aspects. *Rev. Inorg. Chem.,* 2015, *35*, pp 179-189.

[4] Hofmann P., Heiss H., Müller G., Synthesis and Molecular Structure of Dichloro[?/2bis(di-/-butylphosphino)methane]platinum(II), Pt (dtbpm)Cl2. The Electronic Structure of 1,3-Diphosphaplatina cyclobutane Fragments. *Z. Naturforsch.,* 1987, *42b*, pp 395-409.

[5] Babai A., Deacon G. B., Erven A. P., Meyer G., Molecular and Crystal Structures of Pentafluorophenyl-platinum(II) Complexes with Bis(diphenylphosphino)methane, Bis(diphenylarsino)methane and 1,2-Bis(diphenylarsino)ethane *Z. Anorg. Allg. Chem*., 2006, *632,* pp 639-644.

[6] Braun L., Liptau P., Kehr G., Ugolotti J., Frohlich R., Erker G., Bis(diphenylphosphino)acetonitrile: Synthesis, ligand properties and application in catalytic carbon–carbon coupling. *Dalton Trans*., 2007, pp 1409-1415.

[7] Dossett S. J., Gillon A., Orpen A. G., Fleming J. S., Pringle P. G., Wass D. F., Jones M. D., Steric activation of chelate catalysts: efficient polyketone catalysts based on four-membered palladium(II) diphosphine chelates. *Chem. Commun.,* 2001, pp 699-700.

[8] Liang H., Nischide K., Ito S., Yoshifuji M., Preparation, properties, and catalytic activity of transition-metal complexes containing a ligated 2-methyl-3,3-diphenyl-1,3-diphosphapropene skeleton. *Tetrahedron Lett*., 2003, *44*, pp 8297-8300.

[9] Browning C. S., Farrar D. H., Frankel D. C., Structures of $Pd[(PPh_2)_2(NMe)]Cl_2$, $Pt[(PPh_2)_2(NMe)]Cl_2$ and $Pt[(PPh_2)_2(NMe)](CN)_2$. *Acta Crystallogr., Sec. C*, 1992, *48*, pp 806-811.

[10] Clocte N., Visser H. G., Roodt A., [*N,N*-Bis(diphenyl-phosphino)propylamine-κ^2 *P,P'*]dichloridoplatinum(II). *Acta Crystallogr., Sect. E, Struct. Rep. Online*, 2010, *66*, pp m51-m52.

[11] Slawon A. M. Z., Milton H. L., Wheatley J., Woollins J. D., Preparation and coordination chemistry of N-diallylaminodiphenyl phosphine and N-allylaminobis(diphenyl) phosphine. *Polyhedron*, 2004, *23*, pp 3125-3132.

[12] Biricik N., Durap F., Kayan C., Gumgum B., Gurbuz N., Oždemir I., Ang W. H., Tei Z., Scopelliti R., Synthesis of new aminophosphine

complexes and their catalytic activities in C–C coupling reactions. *J. Organomet. Chem.,* 2008, *693*, pp 2693-2699.

[13] Gallo V., Mastronilli P., Nobile G.F., Braunstein P., Englert U., Chelating *versus* bridging bonding modes of N-substituted bis(diphenylphosphanyl) amineligands in Pt complexes and Co_2Pt clusters., *Dalton Trans.,* 2006, pp 2342-2349.

[14] Slawin A. M. Z., Woollins J. D., Zhang Q., Novel chiral phosphine ligands and complexes from amino acid esters. *J. Chem. Soc., Dalton Trans.,* 2001, pp 621-632.

[15] Calabro G., Drommi D., Graiff C., Faraone F., Tiripiccio A., Rhodium(I), Palladium(II) and Platinum(II) Coordination Chemistry of the Short-Bite Chiral Ligands (Sc)-N,N-Bis(diphenylphosphanyl)-sec-butylamine, (Ra,Ra)-N,N-Bis(binaphthylphosphonito) phenyl-amine and (Ra,Sc)-N-(Diphenylphosphanyl)-N-(binaphthylphos phonito)-sec-butylamine. Eur. J. Inorg. Chem., 2004, pp 1447-1453.

[16] Tei Z., Scopelliti R., Dyson P. J., On the Reactivity of the Iminodiphosphane $C_6H_4(o\text{-CN})N{=}PPh_2{-}PPh_2$: Fragmentation Versus Isomerisation. *Eur. J. Inorg. Chem.,* 2004, pp 530-537.

[17] Tei Z., Ang W. H., Zhao D., Scopelliti R., Dyson P. J., Complexation associated rearrangement of iminobiphosphines to diphosphino amines. *Inorg. Chim. Acta*, 2006, *359*, pp 2635-2643.

[18] Durap F., Biricik N., Gumgum B., Ozkar S., Ang W. H., Tei Z., Scopelliti, R., Synthesis and characterizations of N,N-bis(diphenylphosphino)ethylaniline derivatives and X-ray crystal structure of palladium (II), platinum (II) complexes. *Polyhedron*, 2008, *27*, pp 196-202.

[19] Aydemir M., Durap F., Baysal A., Akba O., Gumgum B., Ozkar S., Yildirim L. T., Synthesis and characterization of new bis(diphenylphosphino)aniline ligands and their complexes: X-ray crystal structure of palladium(II) and platinum(II) complexes, and application of palladium(II) complexes as pre-catalysts in Heck and Suzuki cross-coupling reactions. *Polyhedron*, 2009, *28*, pp 2313-2320.

[20] Gaw K. G., Smith M. B., Wright J. B., Slawin A. M. Z., Coles S. J., Hursthouse M. B., Tizzard G. J., Square-planar metal(II) complexes

containing ester functionalised bis(phosphino)amines: Mild P−N methanolysis and Carene−H cyclometallation. *J. Organomet. Chem.*, 2012, *699*, pp 39-47.

[21] Biricik N., Duarp F., Gumgum B., Tei Z., Scopelliti R., Synthesis and reactivity of *N,N-bis*(diphenylphosphino)dimethylaniline compounds. *Transition Met. Chem.*, 2007, *32*, pp 877-883.

[22] Aydamir M., Baysal A., Sahin E., Gumgum B., Ozkar S., Aminophosphine–palladium(II) complexes: Synthsesis, structure and applications in Suzuki and Heck cross-coupling reactions. *Inorg. Chim. Acta*, 2011, *378*, pp 10-18.

[23] Al-Masrá H. T., Synthesis, Characterization, and Structures of Palladium(II) and Platinum(II) Complexes Containing *N,N*-Bis(diphenylphosphanyl)Naphthylamine. *Z. Anorg. Allg. Chem.*, 2012, *638*, pp 1012-1017.

[24] Ferrer M., Rossell O., Ruiz E., Maestro M. A., Equilibria between Metallosupramolecular Squares and Triangles with the New Rigid Linker 1,4-Bis(4-pyridyl)tetrafluorobenzene. Experimental and Theoretical Study of the Structural Dependence of NMR Data. *Inorg. Chem.*, 2003, *42*, pp 5890-5899.

[25] Gunay A., Brennessel W. W., Jones W. D., A second polymorph of [1,2-bis(di-*tert*-butylphosphino)ethane]dichloridoplatinum(II). *Acta Crystallogr., Sect. E, Struct. Rep. Online*, 2008, *64*, pp m454.

[26] Harada M., Kai Y., Yasuoka N., Kasai N., The Crystal and Molecular Structures of Dichloro-1,2-bis(di-*t*-butylphosphino)ethaneplatinum (II) and its Chlorobenzene Solvate. *Bull. Chem. Soc. Jpn.*, 1976, *49*, pp 3472-3477.

[27] Farrar D. H., Ferguson G., The crystal and molecular structure of dichloro-(bis-1,2-diphenylphosphinoethane)platinum(II). *J. Crystallogr. Spectr. Res.*,1982, *12,* pp 465-471.

[28] Engelhardt L. M., Patrick J. M., Raston C. L., Turis P., White A. H., Crystal structures of Bis[(ethane-1,2-diyl)bis(diphenylphosphine)]-palladium(II) and -platinum(II) dichloride dichloromethane and Dichloro[(ethane-1,2-diyl)bis(diphenylphosphine)]platinum(II) dichloromethane. *Aust. J. Chem.*, 1984, *37*, pp 2193-2200.

[29] Oberhausser W., Bachmann C., Brüggeller P., Palladium (II) and platinum (II) complexes of cis-1,2-bis(diphenylphosphino)ethene: completely planar structures due to π bonding in the case of platinum (II). *Inorg. Chim. Acta.*, 1995, *238*, pp 35-43.

[30] Oberhausser W, Bachmann C., Stampfl T., Haid R., Langes C., Rieder A., Brüggeller P., Nickel(II), palladium(II), platinum(II) and platinum(IV) complexes of cis-1,2-bis(diphenylphosphino) ethene and nitrogen-containing heterocycles or sulfur ligands. *Inorg. Chim. Acta*, 1998, *274*, pp 143-154.

[31] M. Lutz, A. L. Spek, S. H. L. Thoonen, B. J. Deelman, G. van Koten, Crystal and molecular structure of bis(dipenylphosphino)ethane dichloride platinum(II) complex. *Private Communication, (CCDC, DEBUDO 1)* (2002).

[32] Mague J. T., Tink M. J., Recatto C. A., Structure of *cis*-[1,2-bis(di-cyclohexylphosphino)ethane-*P*,*P'*]dichloroplatinum(II) chloroform solvate. *Acta Crystallogr., Sect. C*, 1993, *49*, pp 1176-1178.

[33] Powell J., Horvath M. J., Lough A., Synthesis and structural characterization of [$PtCl_2${*meso*-Ph(HO)PCH_2CH_2P(OH)Ph}] and structurally related derivatives. *J. Chem. Soc., Dalton Trans.*, 1996, pp 1679-1685.

[34] Jones N. D., Meessen P., Losehand U., Patrick B. O., James B. R., Platinum(II) and Palladium(II) Complexes of Bisphosphine Ligands Bearing *o-N,N*-Dimethylanilinyl Substituents: A Hint of Catalytic Olefin Hydration. *Inorg. Chem.*, 2005, *44*, pp 3290-3298.

[35] Dennett J. N. L., Gillon A. L., Heslop K., Hyett D. J., Fleming J. S., Lloyd-Jones C. E., Orpen A. G., Pringle P. G., Wass D. F., Soutt J. N., Wheatherhead R. H., Diphosphine Complexes of Nickel(II) Are Efficient Catalysts for the Polymerization and Oligomerization of Ethylene: Steric Activation and Ligand Backbone Effects. *Organometallics*, 2004, *23*, pp 6077-6079.

[36] Baber A., de Vries J. G., Orpen A. G., Pringle P. G., von der Luche K., Allosteric effects in asymmetric hydrogenationcatalysis? Asymmetric induction as a function of the substrate and the backbone flexibility of C_1-

symmetric diphosphines in rhodium-catalysed hydrogenations. *Dalton Trans*., 2006, pp 4821-4828.

[37] Guino-o M. A., Zureick A. H., Blank N. F., Anderson B. J., Chapp T. W., Kim Y., Glueck D. S., Rheingold A. L., Synthesis and Structure of Platinum Bis(phospholane) Complexes Pt(diphos*)(R)(X), Catalyst Precursors for Asymmetric Phosphine Alkylation. Organometallics, 2012, *31*, pp 6900-6910.

[38] Claver C., Fernandez E., Gillon A. L., Heslop K. M., Hyett D. J., Martorell A., Orpen A. G., Pringle P. G., Biarylphosphonites: a class of monodentate phosphorus(III) ligands that outperform their chelating analogues in asymmetric hydrogenation catalysis. *Chem. Commun*., 2000, pp 961-962.

[39] Johanson M. H., Malmstrom T., Wendt O. F., Chiral platinum(II) complexes. Crystal and molecular structures of cis-[PtPhCl((R,R)-CHIRAPHOS)] and cis-[PtCl2((R,R)-CHIRAPHOS)]. *Inorg. Chim. Acta*, 2001, *316*, pp 149-152.

[40] Yeo, W. Ch., Tan G. K., Koh L. L., Leung P. H., Asymmetric [2+2] Cycloaddition of (*E*)-2-(Diphenylphosphanyl)styrene Promoted by a Chiral Metal Template. *Eur. J. Inorg. Chem*., 2005, pp 4723-4728.

[41] Dahlenburg L., Mertel S., Chiral chelate phosphanes: XI. Application of cyclopentane-based C2 chiral bis(phosphane) ligands C5H8(PR2)2 to Pt□Sn-catalyzed styrene hydroformylation. *J. Organomet. Chem*., 2001, *630*, pp 221-243.

[42] Pullarkat S. A., Cheow Y. L., Li Y., Leung P. H., Enantioselective, High-Yielding Synthesis of Alcohol-Functionalized Diphosphanes Utilizing Asymmetric Control with a Chiral Auxiliary. *Eur. J. Inorg. Chem*., 2009, pp 2375-2382.

[43] Liu F., Pullarkat S. A., Tan K. W., Li Y., Leung P. H., Enantioselective Diels–Alder Reaction of 3-Diphenylphosphinofuran with 1-Phenyl-3,4-dimethylphosphole and Subsequent Synthetic Manipulations of the Cycloadduct. *Organometallics*, 2009, *28*, pp 6254-6259.

[44] Yeo W. Ch., Vittal J. J., Koh L. L., Tan G. K., Leung P. H., Functionalization of Metal-Protected Chiral Phosphines via Simple Organic Transformations. *Organometallics*, 2006, *25*, pp 1259-1269.

[45] Yeo W.Ch., Chen S., Tan G.K., Leung P.H., Synthesis of P-chiral phosphines via chiral metal template promoted asymmetric furan Diels–Alder reaction. *J. Organomet. Chem.*, 2007, *692*, pp 2539-2547.

[46] Smith E. A. S., Molev G., Botoshansky M., Gandelman M., Modifiable bidentate systems *via* N–C rearrangement in triazoles. *Chem. Commun.*, 2011, *47*, pp 319-321.

[47] S. Paavola, F. Teixidor, C. Vinas, R. Kivekas, *cis*-[1,2-Bis(diisopropylphosphino-κ*P*)-1,2-dicarba-*closo*-dodecaborane]dichloroplatinum(II) dichloromethane hemisolvate. *Acta Crystallogr., Sect. C, Cryst. Struct. Commun.*, 2002, 58, m237.

[48] Maulana I., Lonnecke P., Hey-Hawkins E., Platinum(II) and Palladium(II) Complexes of Chiral P−Cl Functionalized Bisphosphino*ortho*-Carbaboranes. *Inorg. Chem.*, 2009, *48*, pp 8638-8645.

[49] Dodds D. L., Haddow M. F., Orpen A. G., Pringle P. G., Woodward G., Stereospecific Diphosphination of Activated Acetylenes: A General Route to Backbone-Functionalized, Chelating 1,2-Diphosphinoethenes. *Organometallics*, 2006, *25*, pp 5937-5945.

[50] Lavery C. B., Ferguson M. J., Stradiotto M., Platinum-Catalyzed Alkene Cyclohydroamination: Evaluating the Utility of Bidentate P,N/P,P Ligation and Phosphine-Free Catalyst Systems. *Organometallics*, 2010, *29*, pp 6125-6128.

[51] Liu S. T., Chen J. T., Peng S. M., Hsiao Y. L., Cheng M. Ch, Structural analysis of o-phenylenebis(diisopropylphosphine) complexes of nickel(II), palladium(II), and platinum(II). *Inorg. Chem.*, 1990, *29*, pp 1169-1172.

[52] Miller P. W., Long N. J., White A. J. P., Synthesis, characterisation and coordination chemistry of a new multidentate P_2N_4 ligand system. *Dalton Trans.*, 2009, pp 5284-5286.

[53] Basra S., de Vries J. G., Heytt D. J., Harrison G., Heslop K. M., Orpen A. G., Pringle P. G., von der Luche K., Efficient asymmetric hydrogenation with rhodium complexes of C_1-symmetric 2,5-dimethylphospholane-diphenylphosphines. *Dalton Trans.*, 2004, pp 1901-1905.

[54] Das A. K., Bulak E., Sarkar B., Lissner F., Schleid T., Niemeyer M., Fiedler J., Kaim W., Structures and Redox Properties of Metal Complexes of the Electron-Deficient Diphosphine Chelate Ligand *R,R*-QuinoxP. *Organometallics*, 2008, *27*, pp 218-223.

[55] Hunt S. W., Wang X., Richmond M. G., Synthesis, reactivity investigation, and X-ray diffraction structures of new platinum(II) compounds containing redox-active diphosphine ligands *J. Mol. Struct.*, 2009, *919*, pp 34-40.

[56] Hunt S. W., Yang L., Wang X., Nesterov V., Richmond M. G., New Pt(II)(dithiolate) Compounds Possessing an Energetically Accessible Diphosphine-Based LUMO: Syntheses, Redox Properties, and Solid-State Structures of $PtCl_2$(pbpcd), Pt(tdt)(pbpcd), and Pt(tdt)(bpcd). *J. Inorg. Organomet. Polym. Mater.*, 2010, *20*, pp 457-467.

[57] Burck S., Hajdok I., Nieger M., Bubrin D., Schulze S., Gudat D., Activation of Polarized Phosphorus-Phosphorus Bonds by Alkynes: Rational Synthesis of Unsymmetrical 1,2-Bisphosphine Ligands and Their Complexes. *Z. Naturforsch., B. Chem. Sci.*, 2009, *64*, pp 63-72.

[58] Gouygai M., Tissot O., Daran J. C., Balaviole G. G. A., Biphosphole: A C_2 Symmetry Chiral Bidentate Ligand. Synthesis and Characterization of Nickel, Palladium, Platinum, and Rhodium Complexes. *Organometallics*, 1997, *16*, pp 1008-1015.

[59] Wicht D. K., Zhuravel M. A., Gregush R. V., Glueck D. S., Gusei I. A., Liable-Sands L. M., Rheingold A. L., Platinum(0) Complexes of Chiral Diphosphines: Enantioface-Selective Binding of *trans*-Stilbene. *Organometallics*, 1998, *17*, pp 1412-1419.

[60] Nakajima Y., Nakatani M., Hayashi K., Shiraishi Y., Takita R., Okazaki M., Ozawa F., Synthesis and structures of platinum diphenylacetylene and dithiolate complexes bearing diphosphinidenecyclobutene ligands (DPCB-Y). *New J. Chem.*, 2010, *34*, pp 1713-1722.

[61] Sreenivasa Reddy V., Katti K. V., Barnes C. L., Transition Metal Chemistry of Main Group Hydrazides, 9. Platinum Complexes of Diphosphanylhydrazides $R_2PN(Me)N(Me)PR_2 \cdot PtCl_2$ (R = OPh, *o*-$OC_6H_4CH_2CHCH_2$). *Chem. Ber.*, 1994, *127*, pp 1355-1357.

[62] Schaffer D. J., Batsanov A. S., Jensen C. M., Takara S., Syntheses and crystal structures of a series of palladium(II) and platinum(II) complexes bearing new hydrazine-based bisphosphinite ligands equipped with pyridyl arms. *Polyhedron*, 2010, *29*, pp 1660-1666.

[63] Takara S., Batsanov A. S., Schaffer D. J., Takase M., Kunishige J. A., Lee S. J., Solid-State Structures of *trans*-[$RuCl_2\{Cl_2PN(Me)N(Me)PCl_2\}_2$] and *cis*-[$MCl_2\{Cl_2PN(Me)N(Me)PCl_2\}$] (M = Pt^{II} and Pd^{II}) Studied by X-ray Crystallography and ^{13}C CPMAS NMR Spectroscopy. *Bull. Chem. Soc. Jpn.*, 2007, *80*, pp 1776-1779.

[64] Eberhardt L., Armspach D., Matt D., Oswald B., Toupet L., Efficient asymmetric hydrogenation of olefins with hydrazine-derived diphosphoramidites. *Org. Biomol. Chem.*, 2007, *5*, pp 3340-3346.

[65] Slawin A. M. Z., Wainwright M., Woollins J. D., The preparation and coordination chemistry of phosphorus(III) derivatives of dialkyl hydrazines. *J. Chem. Soc., Dalton Trans.*, 2002, pp 513-519.

[66] Aluri B. R., Peulecke N., Muller B. H., Peitz S., Spannenberg A., Hapke M., Rosenthal U., Synthesis, Coordination Chemistry, and Catalysis of the First 1,2-Bis(diphenylphosphino)-1,2-diphenylhydrazine, $Ph_2PN(Ph)N(Ph)PPh_2$. Organometallics, 2010, *29*, pp 226-231.

[67] Brown G. M., Elsegood M. R. J., Smith M. B., Blann K., Metal(II) template assisted syntheses of two P—C—O—P chelating ligands incorporating a bulky 1,3,5,7-tetramethyl-2,4,8-trioxa-6-phospha-adamantyl cage. *Inorg. Chem. Commun.*, 2011, *14*, pp 940-943.

In: New Developments in Oncology Research ISBN: 978-1-53615-365-1
Editor: Marcos T. Blair
© 2019 Nova Science Publishers, Inc.

Chapter 5

ORGANODIPHOSPHINES IN CIS – PT(η^2-PXXXP)CL$_2$ DERIVATIVES: STRUCTURAL ASPECTS

Milan Melník, Andrea Forgacsova and Peter Mikuš
Department of Pharmaceutical Analysis and Nuclear Pharmacy, Faculty of Pharmacy, Comenius University in Bratislava, Bratislava, Slovak Republic
Toxicological and Antidoping Center, Faculty of Pharmacy, Comenius University in Bratislava, Bratislava, Slovak Republic

ABSTRACT

This review includes over forty cis-Pt(η^2-PXXXP)Cl$_2$ derivatives in which organodiphosphines create six-membered metallocyclic rings. There are wide varieties of the respective rings of the types: PC$_3$P (most common), PCNCP, PCSCP, PCSiCP, PNCNP, PCCOP, PCCNP, POPNP, POSiOP and P(XXX)$_2$P. The total mean values of Pt-P and Pt-Cl bond distances are 2.222 Å and 2.358 Å. The total mean values of the bite P-Pt-P bond angles is 94.0°. These data are compared and discussed with those found in cis-PtP_2Cl_2 derivatives of $Pt(\eta^2\text{-}PXP)(Cl)_2$ and $Pt(\eta^2\text{-}PX_2P)(Cl)_2$ types. There are complexes which are examples of distortion isomerism.

Keywords: structure, cis-PtP_2Cl_2, organodiphosphine, six-membered chelate rings, isomers

ABBREVIATIONS

$Bu^t_2P(C_7H_6)PBu^t_2$	di-t-butyl(2-di-t-utylphoshino)benzyl)phosphine
$Bu^t_2P(C_7H_6)P(\eta^2\text{-}C_{10}H_{14}O_3)$	8-(2-((di-t-butylphosphino)methyl)phenyl)-1,3,5,7-tetramethyl-2,4,6-trioxa-8-phosphatricyclo [3.3.1.1^{3,7}]decane
$(\eta^2\text{-}C_4H_8)P(CH_2)_3P(\eta^2\text{-}C_4H_8)$	1,1'-(1,3-propanediyl)bisphospholane
$(\eta^2\text{-}C_5H_{10})P(CH_2)_3P(\eta^2\text{-}C_5H_{10})$	1,1'-(1,3-propanediyl)bisphosphinane
$(\eta^2\text{-}C_{10}H_{10})P(CH_2)_3P((\eta^2\text{-}C_{10}H_{12})$	1,1'-(1,3-propanediyl)bisphosphenane
$(C_{12}H_4F_{13})_2P(CH_2)_3P(C_{12}H_4F_{13})_2$	propane-1,3-diylbis(bis(4-(tridecafluorohexyl) phenyl)phosphine
$MesP(CH_2N(C_8H_5O_4)CH_2)_2PMes$	3,7-(1,5-bis(3,5-dicarboxylphenyl)-3,7-bis(mesityl)-1,5-diaza-3,7-diphosphacyclooctane)
$Ph_2P((CH_2SCH_2)PPh_2$	((sulfanediylbis(methylene))bis(diphenylphosphine)
$Ph_2P(C_{10}H_6)PPh_2$	naphtalene-1,8-diylbis(diphenylphosphine)
$Ph_2P(C_5H_5)PPh_2$	bis(diphenylphosphino)pentane-2,4-diyl
$Ph_2P(C_5H_8O)PPh_2$	bis(diphenylphosphino)-2-ethyl-3-oxapropane
$Ph_2P(C_5H_8O_2)Ph_2$	2,2-bis(diphenylphosphinomethyl)propionic acid
$Ph_2P(C_5H_9N)PPh_2$	1-diphenylphosphino-2-(diphenylphosphinomethyl) pyrrolidine

$Ph_2P(C_5H_9PPh_2)PPh_2$	1,1,1-tris(diphenylphosphinomethyl)ethane
$Ph_2P(C_6H_4)PPh_2$	bis(diphenylphosphino)cyclohexyl
$Ph_2P(C_6H_6O)PPh_2$	3,5-bis(diphenylphosphino)-7-oxabicyclo[2.2.1]hept-2-ene
$Ph_2P(C_7H_6N_4)PPh_2$	(diphenylphosphino(5-(diphenylphosphino)pyrazolyl) pyrazolyl)methane
$Ph_2P(CH_2)_3P(\eta^2\text{-}C_6H_{12})$	1-((2'R,5'R)-2',5'-dimethylphospholano)-3-(diphenylphosphino)propane
$Ph_2P(CH_2CH(CH_2OH)O)PPh_2$	3-(diphenylphosphanyl)-2-((diphenylphosphonito) propanol
$(Ph_2PCH_2)(Ph)P(CH_2)_3P(Ph)(CH_2PPh_2)$	P,P'-bis(diphenylphosphinomethyl)-P,P'-diphenylpropane-1,3-diphospine
$Ph_2P(CH_2N(C_4H_8SePh)CH_2)PPh_2$	N,N-bis((diphenylphosphino)methyl)-N-(4-(phenylseleno)butyl)amine
$Ph_2P(CH_2N(C_7H_7O)CH_2)PPh_2$	(N,N-bis(diphenylphosphino)methyl-4-methoxyaniline
$Ph_2P(CH_2N(Ph)CH_2)P(\eta^2\text{-}C_{10}H_{16}O_3)$	1,3,5,7-tetramethyl-6-(N-(diphenylphosphanyl-methyl)-N-(phenyl)aminomethyl)-2,4,8-trioxa-6-phosphaadamantane
$Ph_2P(CH_2N(Ph)CH_2)PPh_2$	(N,N-bis(diphenylphosphino)methyl)aniline
$Ph_2P(CH_2Si(Me)_2CH_2)PPh_2$	2,2-dimethyl-1,3-bis(diphenylphosphino)-2-silapropane
$Ph_2P(N(Me)C(=O)N(Me))PPh_2$	N,N'-dimethyl-N,N'-bis(diphenylphosphino)urea
$Pr^i_2P(C_{12}H_8)P(H)(Ph)$	diisopropyl(6-phenylphosphino)-1,2-dihydroacenaphthylen-5-yl)phosphine

1. INTRODUCTION

The chemistry of platinum is particularly important in the areas of catalysis and biochemistry. In our previous reviews we dealt with four-coordinate PtP_2Cl_2 derivatives (260 examples) in which organomonodentate –P donor ligands were involved [1] and over 85 examples in which organodiphosphine –P,P' donor ligands were involved formed four- and five- membered metallocyclic rings [2]. This review presents a brief survey of the square- planar PtP_2Cl_2 derivatives in which organodiphosphines –P,P donor ligands are involved which form a six- membered metallocyclic rings. The primary source of the information has been Cambridge Crystallographic Database.

2. Cis-Pt(H²-PXXXP)Cl₂ Derivatives

There are over forty examples in which each Pt(II) atom has a square-planar environment with varying degrees of distortion, build up by organodiphosphine -P,P'- donor ligands and a pair of chlorine atoms. The homodiphosphine ligands create wide variety of the atoms between the P,P'-donor atoms. These varieties are: PC_3P (24 examples), PCNCP (6 examples), PCSCP (1 example), PCSiCP (1 example), PNCNP (3 examples), POSiOP (1 example), POPNP (1 example), PC_2OP (1 example), and PC_2NP (1 example). There are even examples in which organodiphosphines create twin chelate rings of the type: $P(CNC)_2P$ (3 examples) and P(CNC)(CCC)P (1 example).

2.1. Cis-Pt(η^2-PC_3P)(Cl)₂ Type

There are twenty four examples of this type which crystallize in the three crystal systems: triclinic (3 examples), orthorhombic (8 examples) and monoclinic (thirteen examples).

Such complexes are: [Pt{η^2-$Bu^t_2(CH_2)_3PBu^t_2$}$(Cl)_2$].0.5(PhCl) [3],[Pt{η^2-$Ph_2P(CH_2)_3PPh_2$}$(Cl)_2$] [4], [Pt{η^2-$Ph_2P(CH_2)_3PPh_2$}$(Cl)_2$]. 0.5 (C_6H_6) [5}, [Pt{η^2-$Ph_2P(CH_2)_3PPh_2$}$(Cl)_2$].CH_2Cl_2 [6, 7], [Pt{η^2-$cy_2P(CH_2)_3Pcy_2$}$(Cl)_2$].2CH_2Cl_2 [8], [Pt{η^2-(η^2-C_4H_8)$P(CH_2)_3P$(η^2-C_4H_8)} $(Cl)_2$]$CHCl_3$ [9], [Pt{η^2-(η^2-C_5H_{10})$P(CH_2)_3P$(η^2-C_5H_{10})}$(Cl)_2$] [9], [Pt{η^2-

$(\eta^2$-$C_6H_{12})P(CH_2)_3P(\eta^2$-$C_6H_{12})\}(Cl)_2]$ [9], $[Pt\{\eta^2$-$(C_{12}H_4F_{13})_2P(CH_2)_3P(C_{12}H_4F_{13})_2\}(Cl)_2]$ [10], $[Pt\{\eta^2$-$(Ph_2P(CH_2)(Ph)P(CH_2)_3P(Ph)(CH_2PPh_2)\}(Cl)_2].H_2O$ [11], $[Pt\{\eta^2$-$Ph_2P(CH_2)_3P(\eta^2$-$C_6H_{12})\}(Cl)_2]$ [12], $[Pt\{\eta^2$-$Ph_2P(C_6H_4)PPh_2\}(Cl)_2]$ [13], $[Pt\{\eta^2$-$Ph_2P)(C_5H_8O)PPh_2\}(Cl)_2]$ [13], $[Pt\{\eta^2$-$Ph_2P(C_5H_5)PPh_2\}(Cl)_2$ [14], $[Pt\{\eta^2$-$Ph_2P(C_5H_8O_2)PPh_2\}(Cl)_2]Me_2SO$ [15], $[Pt\{\eta^2$-$Ph_2P(C_6H_6O)PPh_2\}(Cl)_2]$ [16], $[Pt\{\eta^2$-$Ph_2P(C_{10}H_6)PPh_2\}(Cl)_2].CH_2Cl_2$ [17], $[Pt\{\eta^2$-$(Ph)(Bu^t)P(C_{10}H_6)P(Bu^t)(Ph)\}(Cl)_2].CH_2Cl_2$ [18], $[Pt\{\eta^2$-$(C_6F_5)(Me)P(C_{10}H_6)P(Me)(C_6F_5)\}(Cl)_2].CH_2Cl_2$ [18], $[Pt\{\eta^2$-$Bu^t{}_2P(C_7H_6)PBu^t{}_2(Cl)_2].CH_2Cl_2$ [19], $[Pt\{\eta^2$-$Bu^t{}_2P(C_7H_6)P(\eta^2$-$C_{10}H_{14}O_3)\}(Cl)_2].CH_2Cl_2$ [19], $[Pt\{\eta^2$-$Pr^i{}_2P(C_{12}H_8)P(H)(Ph)\}(Cl)_2]$ [20], $[Pt\{\eta^2$-$Ph_2P(C_6H_2F_6O)PPh_2\}(Cl)_2]$ [21], and $[Pt\{\eta^2$-$Ph_2P(C_5H_9PPh_2)PPh_2\}(Cl)_2]$ [22]. Structure of $[Pt\{\eta^2$-$Bu^t{}_2P(C_7H_6)PBu^t{}_2(Cl)_2].CH_2Cl_2$ [19] is shown in Figure 1 as an example. The mean value of P-Pt-P bite angle is 94.6° (PC_3P).

2.2. Cis-$Pt(\eta^2$-PCXCP)$(Cl)_2$ (X = N, S or Si) Type

There are six examples of the cis-$Pt(\eta^2$-PCNCP)$(Cl)_2$ type. These complexes crystallized in three crystal systems: orthorhombic (one example), triclinic (one example) and monoclinic (four examples). Such complexes are: $[Pt\{\eta^2$-$Ph_2P(CH_2N(Ph)CH_2)PPh_2\}(Cl)_2].CHCl_3$ [23], $[Pt\{\eta^2$-$Ph_2P(CH_2N(C_7H_7O)CH_2)PPh_2\}(Cl)_2].CH_2Cl_2$ [24], $[Pt\{\eta^2$-$Ph_2P(CH_2N(Ph)CH_2)P(\eta^2$-$C_{10}H_{16}O_3)\}(Cl)_2].CHCl_3$ [25], $[Pt\{\eta^2$-$Ph_2P(CH_2N(p$-$tolyl)CH_2)P(\eta^2$-$C_{10}H_{16}O_3)\}(Cl)_2].CHCl_3.Et_2O$ [25], $[Pt\{\eta^2$-$Ph_2P(CH_2N(C_4H_8SePh)CH_2)PPh_2\}(Cl)_2]$ [26], and $[Pt\{\eta^2$-$Ph_2P(C_7H_6N_4)PPh_2\}(Cl)_2].CH_2Cl_2$ [27]. Structure of $[Pt\{\eta^2$-$Ph_2P(CH_2N(C_7H_7O)CH_2)PPh_2\}(Cl)_2].CH_2Cl_2$ [24] is shown in Figure 2 as an example. The mean value of P-Pt-P bite angle is 94.0° (PCNCP).

Monoclinic $[Pt\{\eta^2$-$Ph_2P(CH_2SCH_2)PPh_2\}(Cl)_2]$ [23] is only example in which homobidentate –P,P donor ligand creates six-membered metallocyclic ring of the PCSCP type (95.8°).

Orthorhombic $[Pt\{\eta^2$-$Ph_2P(CH_2Si(Me)_2CH_2)PPh_2\}(Cl)_2]$ [28] is also only example of the PCSiCP metallocyclic ring (96.8°).

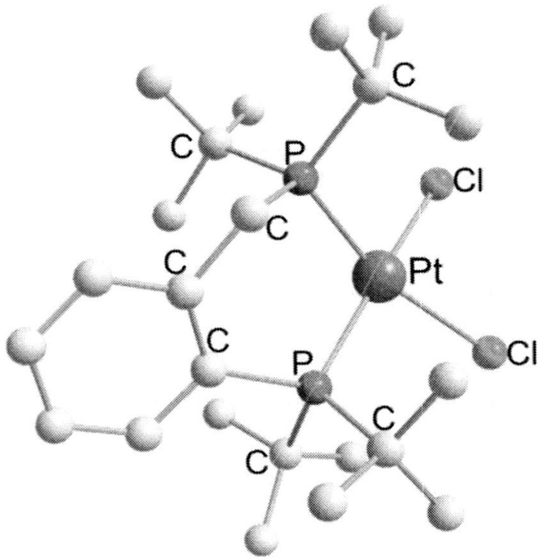

Figure 1. Structure of [Pt{η^2-$Bu^t_2P(C_7H_6)PBu^t_2(Cl)_2$] [19].

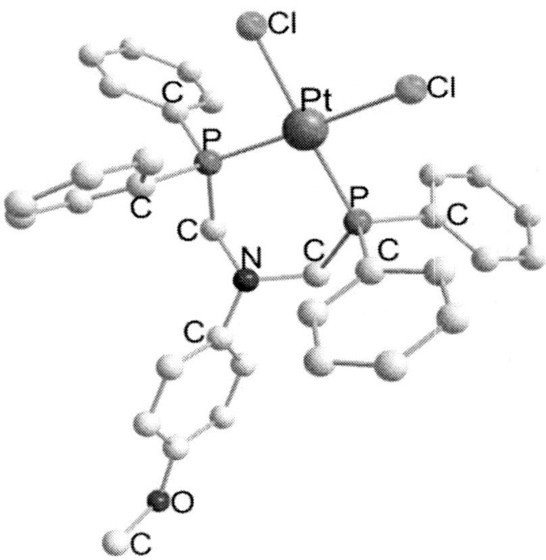

Figure 2. Structure of [Pt{η^2-$Ph_2P(CH_2N(C_7H_7O)CH_2)PPh_2$}$(Cl)_2$] [24].

2.3. Cis-Pt(η^2-PNCNP)$(Cl)_2$ Type

There are three examples, monoclinic [Pt{η^2-Ph_2P(N(Me)C(=O)N(Me)PPh_2}$(Cl)_2$] [29], triclinic [Pt{η^2-Ph_2P(N(Et))C(=O)N(Et))PPh_2}$(Cl)_2$] [29] and orthorhombic [Pt{η^2-Ph_2P(N(Me)C(=O)N(Me)PPh_2}$(Cl)_2$]. $CHCl_3$ [30] in which the chelating -P,P' donor ligands create six- membered metallocyclic rings of the PNCNP type. Structure of [Pt{η^2-Ph_2P(N(Me)C(=O)N(Me)PPh_2}$(Cl)_2$] [29] is shown in Figure 3 as an example. The mean value of the P-Pt-P bite angle is 94.0° (PNCNP).

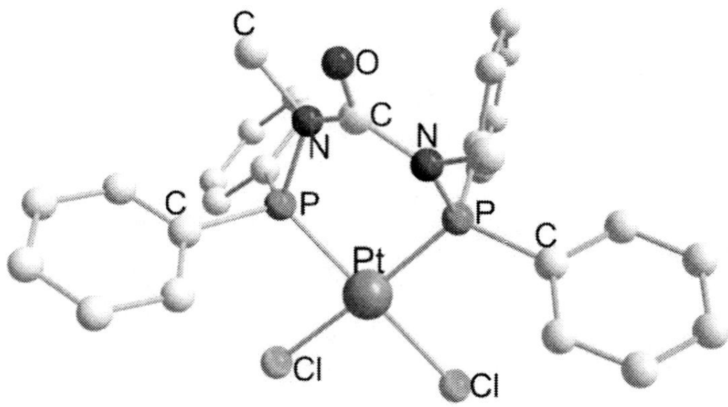

Figure 3. Structure of [Pt{η^2-Ph_2P(N(Me)C(=O)N(Me)PPh_2}$(Cl)_2$] [29].

2.4. Cis-(Pt(η^2-PCCXP)/Cl)$_2$ (X = O or N) Type

Orthorhombic [Pt{η^2-Ph_2P(CH_2CH(CH_2OH)O))PPh_2}$(Cl)_2$].Et_2O [31] is only example in which chelate -P,P' donor ligand creates six-membered metallocyclic ring of the PCCOP type with the value of P-Pt-P bite angle of 96.5°.

In two monoclinic [Pt{η^2-Ph_2P(C_5H_9N)PPh_2}$(Cl)_2$].toluene [32] and [Pt{η^2-Ph_2P(C_6H_5N)PPh_2}$(Cl)_2$].Me_2SO.$CHCl_3$ [33] the chelating ligands create bite angles of PCCNP type. The former example contains two crysallographically independent molecules within the same crystal; differ mostly by degree of distortion. The mean value of the P-Pt-P bite angle is 95.7°.

2.5. Cis-Pt(η^2-POPNP)(Cl)$_2$ Type

Monoclinic [Pt{η^2-$Ph_2P(OP(Ph_2)N)PPh_2$}$(Cl)_2$]$(Cl)_2$ [34] is only example in which the chelating –P,P' donor ligand creates six-membered metallocyclic ring of the POPNP type with the value of P-Pt-P bite angle of 95.8°. The values of the remaining cis- L-Pt-L bond angles of 88.5° (Cl-Pt-Cl) and 88.0° (P-Pt-Cl, mean). The mean value of trans-P-Pt-Cl bond angles is 173.7°.

2.6. Cis-Pt(η^2-POSiOP)(Cl)$_2$ Type

Monoclinic [Pt{η^2-$Ph_2P(OSi(Ph)_2O)PPh_2$]$(Cl)_2$] [35] is only example in which the chelating -P,P' donor ligand creates six-membered metallocyclic ring (POSiOP) with the value of P-Pt-P bite angle of 96.7°.

2.7. Cis-Pt{η^2-P(XXX)$_2$P}(Cl)$_2$ Type

There are four examples in which the chelating -P,P' donor ligands create a pair of six-membered metallocyclic rings. In monoclinic [Pt{η^2-$PhP(CH_2N(Ph)CH_2)_2PPh$}$(Cl)_2$] [36] and in two triclinic [Pt{η^2-$PhP(CH_2N(C_8H_5O)CH_2)_2PPh$}$(Cl)_2$] [37] and [Pt{$\eta^2$-$Ph_2P(CH_2N(C_8H_5O_4)CH_2)_2PMes$}$(Cl)_2$].dmf [38] the respective chelating -P,P' donor ligands create a pair of P(CNC)$_2$P type with the mean P-Pt-P bite angle of 84.2°.

Structure of monoclinic [Pt{η^2-PhP{$CH_2N(C_8H_5O_4)CH_2$}($CH_2CH_2CH_2$)PPh}$(Cl)_2$].Me_2SO [38] is shown in Figure 4. (Me_2SO) was omitted. As can be seen the chelating -P,P' donor ligand creates a pair of the six-membered rings of P(CNC)(CCC)P type. The values of the P-Pt-P bite angles are 84.5° (CNC) and 85° (CCC), respectively.

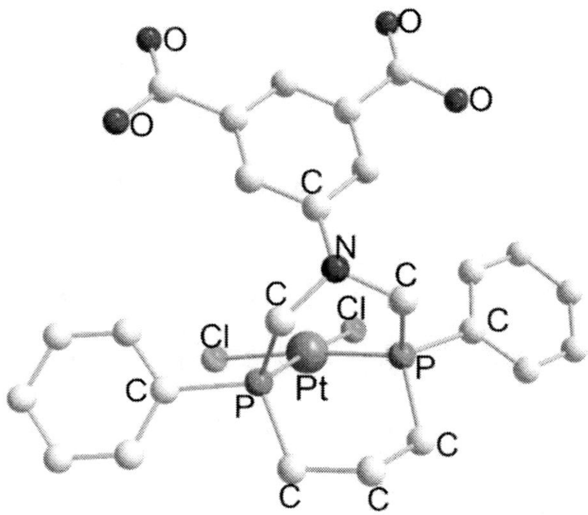

Figure 4. Structure of [Pt{η^2-PhP{$CH_2N(C_8H_5O_4)CH_2$}($CH_2CH_2CH_2$)PPh}$(Cl)_2$] [38].

Conclusion

This review includes over forty cis-PtP_2Cl_2 derivatives in which the chelating -P,P' donor ligands create six-membered metallocyclic rings. There is wide variety of the respective chelate rings of the types: PC_3P (most common), PCNCP, PCSCP, PCSiCP, PNCNP, PCCOP, PCCNP, POPNP, POSiOP and $P(XXX)_2P$. The total mean values of Pt-P and Pt-Cl bond distances are 2.222 Å and 2.358 Å. The total mean values of cis-L-P-L bond angles are: 94.0° (P-Pt-P), 87.6° (Cl-P-Cl) and 89.0° (P-Pt-Cl) and the total mean value of trans-P-Pt-Cl bond angle is 175.3°.

There are two examples [23, 32] which contain two crystallographically independent molecules within the same crystal, differ mostly by degree of distortion and are examples of distortion isomerism [39].

There are cooperative effects between the selected structural parameters in the complexes with four-, five- and six-membered metallocyclic rings (Table 1). As can be seen white P-Pt-P bite angles open with the size of the respective metallocyclic ring, the cis-Cl-Pt-Cl and P-Pt-Cl bond angles closes in the same order. The both Pt-P as well as Pt-Cl bond distances smoothly elongate with the size of the respective chelate rings.

Table 1. Total mean values of selected structural parameters in cis- PtP_2Cl_2 derivatives

Metallocyclic ring (number of examples)	P-Pt-P [°]	Cl-Pt-Cl [°]	P-Pt-Cl [°]	Pt-P [Å]	Pt-Cl [Å]	Pt-L(x4) [Å]
four-membered[a]	72.4	91.7	97.3	2.214	2.352	9.13
(24 examples)				170.4		
five-membered[a]	86.4	88.0	92.7	2.216	2.354	9.14
(31 examples)				175.7		
six-membered	94.0	87.6	89.0	2.222	2.358	9.16
(42 examples)				175.6		

[a]/ ref [2].

ACKNOWLEDGMENTS

This work was supported by the projects VEGA 1/0873/15, KEGA 022UK-4/2015, APVV-15-0585.

REFERENCES

[1] Melník M., Mikuš P., Organomonophosphines in Pt(II) Coordination Complexes. Part I. Monomeric Square Planar (PtP_4, PtP_3X and PtP_2X_2). *Phosphorus, Sulfur, Silicon, Relat. Elem.*, 2015, *190*, pp 1764-1780.

[2] Melník M., Forgácsová A. and Mikuš P., Organodiphosphines in cis-Pt(η^2-PXP)$(Cl)_2$ and cis-Pt(η^2-PXXP)$(Cl)_2$ Derivatives – Structural Aspects. *New Developments in Oncology Research, Nova Science Publ. Inc., NY, USA, 2018, Chapter 1.*

[3] Harada M., Kai Y., Yasuoka N., Kasai N., The Crystal and Molecular Structure of Dichloro[1,3-bis(di-*t*-butylphosphino)propane]platinum (II) Chlorobenzene Solvate. *Bull. Chem. Soc. Jpn.*, 1979, *52*, pp 390-394.

[4] Robertson G. B., Wickramasinghi W. A., *cis*-Di-chloro[tri-methylenebis(diphenylphosphine)]platinum(II). *Acta Crystallogr., Sect. C*, 1987, *43*, pp 1694-1697.

[5] Sivaramakrishna A., Moss J. R., Su H., Novel reactivity aspects of cis-bis(1-alkenyl)platinum(II) compounds of the type Pt(CH2(CH2) nCHCH2)2L2 (where L2=dppp, dppe, dppm and n=1, 2). *Inorg. Chim. Acta*, 2010, *363*, pp 3345-3350.

[6] Deacon G. B., Elliott P. W., Erven A. P., Meyer G., The Synthesis by Decarboxylation Reactions and Crystal Structures of 1, n–Bis (diphenylphosphino)alkane(pentafluorophenyl)-platinum(II) Complexes. *Z. Anorg. Allg. Chem.*, 2005, *631,* pp 843-850.

[7] Kaim W., Dogan A., Klein A., Zalis S., Complexes of 1,3-Bis(diphenylphosphano)propane (dppp) with Dichloroplatinum(II) and Bis(chlorogold(I)): Intramolecular versus Intermolecular Au^I–Au^I Association of [(μ-dppp)$(AuCl)_2$] in *catena* and *cyclo* Forms. *Z. Anorg. Allg. Chem.*, 2005, *63*, pp 1355-1358.

[8] Nicolas E., le Goff X. F., Bouchonnet S., Mezailles N., Room temperature reversible C–H activation mediated by a Pt(0) center, and stoichiometric biphenyl formation *via* solvent activation. *Chem. Commun.*, 2012, *48*, pp 8350.

[9] Haddow M. F., Middleton M. J., Orpen A. G., Pringle P. G., Pap R., Stereoelectronic effects in a homologous series of bidentate cyclic phosphines. A clear correlation of hydroformylation catalyst activity with ring size. *Dalton Trans.*, 2009, pp 202-209.

[10] Berven B. M., Koutsantonis G. A., Skelton B. W., Trengove R. D., White A. H., Highly fluorous complexes of nickel, palladium and platinum: solubility and catalysis in high pressure CO_2. *Dalton Trans.*, 2011, *40*, pp 4167-4174.

[11] Nakajima T., Kurai S., Noda S., Zouda M., Kure B., Tanase T., Cyclic Trinuclear Rh_2M Complexes (M = Rh, Pt, Pd, Ni) Supported by

meso-1,3-Bis[(diphenylphosphinomethyl)phenylphosphino] propane. *Organometallics*, 2012, *31*, pp 4283-4294.

[12] Baber A., de Vries J. G., Orpen A. G., Pringle P. G., von der Luche K., Allosteric effects in asymmetric hydrogenationcatalysis? Asymmetric induction as a function of the substrate and the backbone flexibility of C_1-symmetric diphosphines in rhodium-catalysed hydrogenations. *Dalton Trans*., 2006, pp 4821-4828.

[13] Miller S. P., Jang M., Lachicotte R. J., Eisenberg R., Hydride complexes of platinum(II) containing unsymmetrical di(phosphine) ligands: synthesis, characterization and evidence for pairwise addition of hydrogen based on parahydrogen induced polarization. *Inorg. Chim. Acta,* 1998, *270*, pp 363-375.

[14] Toth I., Elsevier C. J., de Vries J. G., Bakos J., Smeets W. J. J., Spek A. L., Synthesis of Pt compounds containing chiral (2S,4S) -pentane-2,4-diyl-bis(5H-dibenzo[b]phosphindole) as ligand and their use in asymmetric hydroformylation of styrene derivatives. *J. Organomet. Chem.,* 1997, *540*, pp 15-25.

[15] Zhao Ch. Q., Jennings M. C., Puddephatt R. H., Coordination chemistry of 2,2-bis(diphenylphosphinomethyl)propionic acid. *Inorg. Chim. Acta*, 2008, *361*, pp 3301-3308.

[16] Liu F., Pullarkat S. A., Tan K. W., Li Y., Leung P. H., Organoplatinum Complex Promoted the Asymmetric *Endo*Stereochemically Controlled Diels–Alder Reaction between 3-Diphenylphosphinofuran and Diphenylvinylphosphine. *Inorg. Chem*., 2009, *48*, pp 11394-11398.

[17] Niksch T., Goris H., Friedrich M., Oilunkaniemi R., Laitinen R., Weigand W., Synthesis and Characterisation of 2,2-Bis (hydroxymethyl)-1,3-diselenolato Metal(II) Complexes Bearing Various Phosphanes. *Eur. J. Inorg. Chem*., 2010, pp 74-94.

[18] Karacar A., Freatag M., Jones P. G., Bartsch R., Schumtzler R., Platinum(II) Complexes of P-Chiral 1, 8-Bis(diorganophosphino) naphthalenes; Crystal Structures of dmfppn, *rac*-[$PtCl_2$(dmfppn)], and *rac*-[$PtCl_2$(dtbppn)] (dmfppn = 1, 8-di(methyl-pentafluorophenyl phosphino)naphthalene and dtbppn = 1, 8-di(*tert*-butylphenyl

phosphino)naphthalene). *Z. Anorg. Allg. Chem.*, 2002, *628*, pp 533-544.

[19] Fanjul T., Eastham G. Ficure J., Forrest S. J. K, Haddow M. F., Hamilton A., Pringle P. G., Orpen A. G., Weigh M., Interplay of bite angle and cone angle effects. A comparison between *o*-C_6H_4 (CH_2PR_2)(PR'_2) and*o*-C_6H_4(CH_2PR_2)($CH_2PR'_2$) as ligands for Pd-catalysed ethene hydromethoxycarbonylation. *Dalton Trans.*, 2013, *42*, pp 100-115.

[20] Ray M. J., Slawin A. M. Z., Buhl M., Kilian P., *peri*-Substituted Phosphino-Phosphonium Salts: Synthesis and Reactivity. *Organometallics*, 2013, *32*, pp 3481-3492.

[21] Carty A. J., Jacobson S. E., Taylor N. J., Chieh P. C., Base-induced coupling of acetylenes held proximate to a metal: structures of unsymmetrical diphosphine complexes of platinum(II) containing strong vinyl alcohol–amine hydrogen bonds. *J. Chem. Soc., Dalton Trans.*, 1976, pp 1375-1380.

[22] Sevillano P., Habtemariam A., Seijo M. I. G,, Castineiras A., Parsons S., Garcia M. E., Sadler P. J., Homonuclear PdII and PtII and heteronuclear PdII-AuI and PtII-AuI complexes of a tripod triphosphine ligand: synthesis, characterization and reactions with molecules of biological relevance. *Aust. J. Chem.*, 2000, *53*, pp 635-644.

[23] Stickel M., Maichle-Mossmer C., Wesemann L., Mayer H. A., Bis(phosphinomethyl)phenylamines and bis(phosphinomethyl) sulfides and their reaction with d8-platinum group precursors. *Polyhedron*, 2012, *46,* pp 95-104.

[24] Balint E., Fazekas E., Pongracz P., Kollar L., Drahos L., Holczbauer T., Czugler M., Keglevich G., N-Benzyl and N-aryl bis(phospha-Mannich adducts): Synthesis and catalytic activity of the related bidentate chelate platinum complexes in hydroformylation. *J. Organomet. Chem.*, 2012, *717*, pp 75-82.

[25] Brown G. M., Elsegood M. R. J., Lake A. J., Sanchez-Ballester N. M., Smith M. B., Varley T. S., Blann K., Mononuclear and Heterodinuclear Metal Complexes of Nonsymmetric Ditertiary

Phosphanes Derived from R_2PCH_2OH. *Eur. J. Inorg. Chem.*, 2007, pp 1405-1414.

[26] Durran S., Elsegood M. R. J., Smith M. B., New complexes of functionalised ligands bearing P/N/Se or P_2Se donor sets. *New J. Chem.*, 2002, *26*, pp 1402-1408.

[27] Otero A., Carrillo-Hermovilla F., Terreros P., Exposito T., Rojas S., Fernandez-Balza J., Antinolo A., Lopez-Solera I., Synthesis, Structure and Reactivity of New Late Transition Metal Complexes Bearing Diphosphane Ligands Derived from Bis(pyrazol-1-yl)methane. *Eur. J. Inorg. Chem.*, 2003, pp 3233-3241.

[28] Benito M., Rossell O., Seco M., Muller G., Ordinas J. I., Font-Bardia M., Solans., Palladium and Platinum Units Grafted on the Periphery of Carbosilane Dendrimers. *Eur. J. Inorg. Chem.*, 2002, pp 2477-2487.

[29] Slawin A. M. Z., Wainwright M., Woollins J. D., The preparation and coordination chemistry of phosphorus(III) derivatives of dialkyl ureas andthioureas. *J. Chem. Soc., Dalton Trans.*, 2001 pp 2724-2730.

[30] Jones P. G., Schmutzler R., Vogt R., {*N*-[*tert*-Butyl(phenyl)-phosphino]-*N′*-diphenylphosphino-*N,N′*-dimethylurea-*P,P′*}dichloro-platinum(II) chloroform solvate. *Acta Crystallogr., Sect. E: Struct. Rep. Online*, 2002, *58*, pp m476-m477.

[31] Bergamini P., Bertolasi V., Cattabriga M., Ferretti V., Loprieno U., Mantovani N., Marvelli L., Template Synthesis of Chiral Vicinal Diphosphinites as Their Pt^{II} and Pd^{II} Complexes. *Eur. J. Inorg. Chem.*, 2003, pp 918-925.

[32] Műnzenberg R., Rademacher P., Boese R., Chiral platinum (II) complexes with phosphorus derivatives of the amino acid L-proline. NMR spectroscopic and X-ray structure investigations of the *cis* influence of tertiary phosphorus ligands. *J. Mol. Struct.*, 1998, *444*, pp 77-90.

[33] Aucott S. M., Slawin A. M. Z., Woollins J. D., Synthesis of chelate complexes and the dichalcogen derivatives of the unsymmetrical diphosphine ligand $Ph_2PNHC_6H_4PPh_2$. Molecular structure of $[PtCl_2(Ph_2PNHC_6H_4PPh_2)]\cdot 0.75dmso\cdot 0.75CHCl_3$. *J. Chem. Soc., Dalton Trans.*, 2001, pp 2279-2287.

[34] Slawin A. M. Z., Smith M. B., Woollins J. D., A novel MNOP$_3$ metallocycle. Crystal and molecular structure of cis-[PtCl$_2$Ph$_2$ POP(Ph)$_2$NPPh$_2$-P,P′]. *Polyhedron*, 1997, *16*, pp 1563-1566.

[35] Hogg J. K., James S. L., Orpen A. G., Pringle P. G., Chelating diphos ligands with inorganic backbones. Crystal structure of [PtCl$_2${(PPh$_2$O)$_2$SiPh$_2$}]. *J. Organomet. Chem.*, 1994, *480*, pp C1-C3.

[36] Karasik A. A., Bobrov S. V., Nikonov G. N., Pisarevskii P., Litvinov I. A., Dokuchaev A. S., Struchkov Y. T., Enikeev K. M., Crystal and molecular styructure of monoclinic (N,N-bis(diphenylphosphine) methyl)aniline dichloride platinum(II) complex.*Koord. Khim*, 1995, *21*, Engl. Ed., pp 551-556.

[37] Karasik A. A., Naumov R. N., Balueva A. S., Spiridonova Yu. S., Golodkov O. N., Novikova H. V., Belov G. P., Katsyuba S. A., Vandyukova E. E., Lonnecke P., Hey-Hawkins E., Sinyashin O. G., Synthesis, structure, and transition metal complexes of amphiphilic 1,5-diaza-3,7-diphosphacyclooctanes. *Heteroat. Chem.*, 2006, *17*, pp 499-513.

[38] Karasik A. A., Naumov R. N., Spiridonova Yu. S., Sinyashin O. G., Lonnecke P., Hey-Hawkins E., Synthesis, Molecular Structure and Coordination Chemistry of the First 1-Aza-3,7-diphospha-cyclooctanes. *Z. Anorg. Allg. Chem.*, 2007, *633*, pp 205-210.

[39] Melník M., Holloway C. E., Stereochemistry of platinum coordination compounds. *Coord. Chem. Rev.*, 2006, *250*, pp 2261-2270.

In: New Developments in Oncology Research ISBN: 978-1-53615-365-1
Editor: Marcos T. Blair
© 2019 Nova Science Publishers, Inc.

Chapter 6

ORGANODIPHOSPHINES IN CIS-PT(η^2-PXXXXP)CL$_2$ DERIVATIVES: STRUCTURAL ASPECTS

Milan Melník, Andrea Forgácsová and Peter Mikuš
Department of Pharmaceutical Analysis and Nuclear Pharmacy, Faculty of Pharmacy, Comenius University in Bratislava, Bratislava, Slovak Republic
Toxicological an Antidoping Center, Faculty of Pharmacy, Comenius University in Bratislava, Bratislava, Slovak Republic

ABSTRACT

This review includes over thirty cis-Pt(η^2-PXXXXP)Cl_2 derivatives in which organodihosphines create seven- membered metallocyclic rings. There are five varieties of the respective rings of the types: PC_4P (most common), POC_2OP, PNC_2NP, PSC_2SP and PNC_2OP. The mean values of Pt-P and Pt-Cl bond distances are 2.239 Å and 2.346 Å, respectively. The mean values of cis-L-Pt-L bond angles open in the sequence: 87.3° (Cl-Pt-Cl) < 87.7° (P-Pt-Cl) < 96.8° (P-Pt-P). The mean value of trans-P-Pt-Cl bond angle is 173.5°. These data are compared and discussed with those found in cis-PtP_2Cl_2 derivatives of Pt(η^2-PXP)$(Cl)_2$, Pt(η^2-PXXP)$(Cl)_2$ and

$Pt(\eta^2\text{-}PXXXXP)(Cl)_2$ types. There are complexes which are examples of distortion isomerism.

Keywords: structure, cis-PtP_2Cl_2, organodiphosphines, seven-membered metallocycles, `isomers

ABBREVIATIONS

$Bu_2P(C_8H_8)PPh_2$	dibutyl(2-diphenylphosphino) methyl(benzyl)phosphine
$(\eta^2\text{-}C_4H_{10}N_2)P\{N(Me)(CH_2CH_2)N(Me)\}P(\eta^2\text{-}C_4H_{10}N_2)\}$	bis{(N,N'-dimethylamino ethane) phosphine}-1,2-diaminetriethylamine
$(\eta^2\text{-}C_5H_{10}O_2P\{OCH(COOMe)CH(COOMe)O\}P(\eta^2\text{-}C_5H_{10}O_2)$	(dimethyl-2,3-bis(5,5-dimethyl-1,3,2-dioxaphosphinan-2-yl) oxy)succinate
$(\eta^2\text{-}C_{10}H_{18})P(C_8H_8)P(\eta^2\text{-}C_{10}H_{18})$	2,2'-(1,2-phenylenebis(methylene) bis(5,5,6-trimethyl-2-phosphabicyclo[2.2.2]octane
$(\eta^2\text{-}C_{12}H_{18}O_2)P(NC_5H_9O)P(\eta^2\text{-}C_{12}H_{18}O_2)$	N-(2,2'-biphenoxyphosphino)-2-(2,2'-biphenoxyphosphinolymethyl)pyrrolidine
$(\eta^2\text{-}C_{17}H_{16}NO_2)P\{OCH(Ph)CH(Ph)O\}P(\eta^2\text{-}C_{17}H_{16}NO_2)$	1,2-diphenyl-1,2-bis(5,6-dimethyl-N-phenyl-7-phospha-5-norbomene-2,3-dicarboximide-7-oxy)ethyl

$Et_2NP(\eta^2-N_2)$ $C_9H_9O)_2PNEt_2$	bis(1,2-bis(2-(diethylamino)-1-methyl-4-oxobenzeno(e)-1,3,2$^{\lambda3}$-diazaphosphozinan-2-yl)ethane
$Ph_2P(NC_5H_9O)PPh_2$	(1-(diphenylphosphino)-2-(dipgenylphosphino) oxy)methyl)pyrrolidine
$Ph_2P(C_9H_{12})PPh_2$	bicyclo[2.2.1]hept-5-ene-2,3-diylbismethylene)bis (diphenylphosphine)
$Ph_2P(C_{32}H_{20})PPh_2$	15,15'-bi(16-diphenylphosphino) tetracyclo(6.6.2.0^{2,7}.0^{9,14})hexadeca-2(7),3,5,9 (14),10,12,15-heptenyl
$Ph_2P(C_{24}H_{20})PPh_2$	2,2'-bis(diphenylphosphino)-1,1'-binaphthoyl
$Ph_2P(C_{12}H_8)PPh_2$	2,2'-bis(diphenylphosphino)-1,1'-biphenyl
$Ph_2P\{OCH(Ph)$ $CH(Ph)O\}PPh_2$	1,2-bis(diphenylphosphinooxy)-1,2-diphenylethane
$Ph_2P\{SC(COOMe)$ $C(COOMe)S\}PPh_2$	meso-dimethyl-2,3-bis(diphenylphosphinothio (succinate)
$Ph_2P(C_{12}H_{12}S_2)PPh_2$	2,2'-5,5'-tetramethyl-4,4'-bis(diphenylphosphino)-3,3'-bithiophene
$Ph_2P(CH_2C_7H_8O_2CH_2)$ PPh_2	2,2-dimethyl-4,5-bis(diphenylhosphinomethyl)-1,3-dioxalane
$Ph_2P(C_{20}H_{18})PPh_2$	1,2-bis(α-(diphenylphosphino) benzylidine)cyclohexane
$Ph_2P\{OCC(Et)O\}PPh_2$	1,2-bis(diphenylphosphito)butane
$Ph_2P\{OCH(Ph))$ $CH_2O\}PPh_2$	1,2-bis(diphenylphosphinooxy)ethylbenzene
$Ph_2P(C_6H_{10}O_2)PPh_2$	1,2-bis(diphenylphosphinooxy)cyclohexane
$Ph_2P(C_{24}H_{14})PPh_2$	1,16-bis(diphenylphosphino)tetraphenylene
$Ph_2P(C_{18}H_{22}N_2)PPh_2$	6,6'-bis(diphenylphosphino-N,N,N',N',4,4'-hexa methylbiphenyl-2,2'-diamine

$Ph_2P(C_{20}H_{20}N_2)PPh_2$	3,3'-bis(diphenylphosphino)-5,5',6,6',7,7',8,8'-octahydro-2,2'-binaphtalene
$Pr^i_2P\{N(CH_2Ph)CH_2CH_2N(CH_2Ph)\}PPr^i_2$	N,N'-dibenzyl-N,N'-bis(diizopropyl phosphino)-1,2-ethylendiamine

1. Introduction

Phosphorous donor chiral ligands are very attractive and useful forming wide variability of stereochemistry about central transition metals and platinum is no exception. It should not be to overlook that platinum has played a crucial role with development of many branches of science, even though the amount used have been small reliable platinum crucibles were vital an classical analysis which laid the foundation of modern chemistry. The chemistry of platinum is an important area particularly in the field of biochemistry, catalysis and theory.

Recently, we analyzed structural parameters of monomeric PtP_2Cl_2 derivatives in which P-donor ligands are organomonophosphines [1]. In another two reviews we analyzed structural parameters of monomeric PtP_2Cl_2 derivatives in which P-donor ligands are organodiphosphines which form four- and five-membered metallocyclic rings [2] and six- membered metallocyclic [3]. The aim of this paper is analyze structural parameters of monomeric PtP_2Cl_2 derivatives in which the respective organodiphosphines form seven-membered metallocyclic rings.

2. Cis-PtP_2Cl_2 Derivatives

There are over thirty monomeric Pt(II) complexes with such inner coordination sphere in which organodiphosphines form seven- membered metallocyclic rings. These metallocycles can be divided into the five subgroups: PC_4P, POC_2OP, PNC_2NP, PSC_2SP and PNC_2OP.

2.1. Pt(η^2-PC_4P)Cl_2 Type

This type with seventeen examples is the most common. These complexes crystallized in the three crystal classes: triclinic (3 examples), orthorhombic (7 examples) and monoclinic (7 examples). Pale yellow [Pt{η^2-$Ph_2P(CH_2C_7H_8O_2CH_2)PPh_2$}$(Cl)_2$] exists in two crystal classes: triclinic [4] and orthorhombic [5]. The triclinic complex even contains two crystallographically independent molecules within the same crystal. In each complex the organodiphosphine forms a seven- membered metallocyclic rings with the values of 97° (molecule 1), 96° (molecule 2) and 97.0° (orthorhombic). The Pt(II) atoms have a distorted square- planar environment (PtP_2Cl_2). The mean Pt-L bond distances are: 2.33 Å (L = Cl) and 2.255 Å (P) (molecule 1), 2.35 Å and 2.25 Å (molecule 2) and 2.324 Å and 2.246 Å (orthorhombic). The sum of all four Pt-L bond distances growing in the order: 9.13 Å (orthorhombic) < 9.17 Å (molecule 1) < 9.20 Å (molecule 2), this indicates that inner coordination sphere is less crowded in the given order. These complexes are classical examples of distortion isomerism [6].

In the following fifteen complexes, namely: [Pt{η^2-$Ph_2P(CH_2CH_2CH_2CH_2)PPh_2$}$(Cl)_2$] [7], [Pt{$\eta^2$-$Ph_2P(C_9H_{12})PPh_2$}$(Cl)_2$].$CH_2Cl_2$ (at 233K) [8], [Pt{η^2-$Ph_2P(C_{20}H_{18})$. PPh_2}$(Cl)_2$].4$CHCl_3$ (at 153K) [9], [Pt{η^2-$Bu_2P(C_8H_8)PPh_2$}$(Cl)_2$].CH_2Cl_2 (at 100K) [10], [Pt{η^2-$Bu^t{}_2P(C_8H_8)PPh_2$}$(Cl)_2$]. CH_2Cl_2 (at 100K) [10], [Pt{η^2-$Bu^t{}_2P(C_8H_8)PBu^t{}_2$}$(Cl)_2$].$CHCl_3$ (at 120K) [11], [Pt{η^2-$Ph_2P(C_{32}H_{20})PPh_2$}$(Cl)_2$].2CH_2Cl_2 (at 150K) [12], [Pt{η^2-$Ph_2P(C_{12}H_{18})PPh_2$}$(Cl)_2$].0.5CH_2Cl_2 [13], [Pt{η^2-$Ph_2P(C_{24}H_{20})PPh_2$}$(Cl)_2$] (at 150K) [14], [Pt{η^2-$Ph_2P(C_{12}H_8)PPh_2$}$(Cl)_2$]. CH_2Cl_2 [15], [Pt{η^2-$Ph_2P(C_{24}H_{14})PPh_2$}$(Cl)_2$].2CH_2Cl_2 [16], [Pt{η^2-$Ph_2P(C_{20}H_{20}N_2)PPh_2$}$(Cl)_2$].4$CH_2Cl_2$ (at 150K) [17], [Pt{η^2-$Ph_2P(C_{18}H_{22}N_2)PPh_2$}$(Cl)_2$].2$CH_2Cl_2$ (at 100K) [18], [Pt{η^2-$Ph_2P(C_{12}H_{12}S_2)PPh_2$}$(Cl)_2$] [19], and [Pt{$\eta^2$-($\eta^2$- $C_{10}H_{18})P(C_8H_8)P(\eta^2$-$C_{10}H_{18})$}$(Cl)_2$].$CH_3CN$ (at 150K) [20], each homobidentate –P,P' donor ligands create seven-membered metallocyclic rings of the PC_4P type. Structure of monoclinic [Pt{η^2-$Ph_2P(C_{18}H_{22}N_2)PPh_2$}$(Cl)_2$] [18] is shown in Figure 1 as an example. The mean values of Pt-L bond distances are 2.250 Å (L = P) and 2.335 Å (Cl). The mean values of cis-L-Pt-L bond angles open in the order: 86.8° (Cl-Pt-Cl) < 88.2° (Cl-Pt-P) < 96.7° (P-Pt-P). The mean value of trans-Cl-Pt-P bond angle is 173.2°.

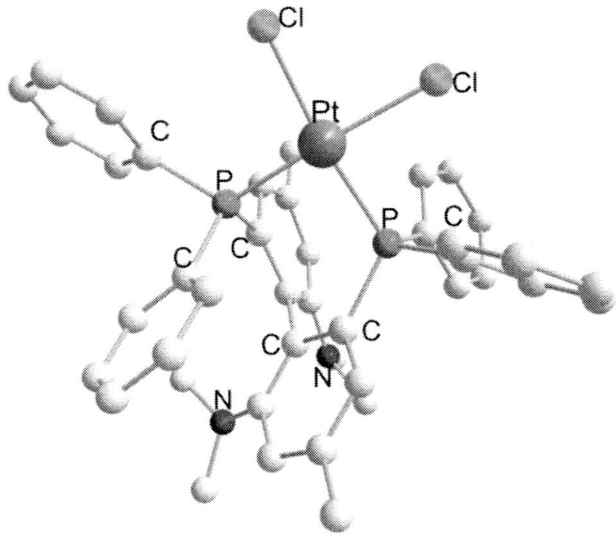

Figure 1. Structure of [Pt{η^2-$Ph_2P(C_{18}H_{22}N_2)PPh_2$}$(Cl)_2$] [18].

2.2. Pt(η^2-POC_2OP)Cl_2 Type

There are six examples of this type. These complexes crystallized in the three crystal classes: orthorhombic (1 example), triclinic (1 example) and monoclinic (4 examples). Such complexes are: [Pt{η^2-Ph_2P{OCC (Et)O}PPh_2}$(Cl)_2$] [21], [Pt{η^2-Ph_2P(OCH(Ph)CH(Ph)O}. $PPh_2(Cl)_2$]. $CHCl_3$ [22], [Pt{η^2-Ph_2P(OCH(Ph)CH_2O}PPh_2}$(Cl)_2$].$CHCl_3$ [22], [Pt{η^2-$Ph_2P(C_6H_{10}O_2)PPh_2$}$(Cl)_2$].CH_2Cl_2 [23], [Pt{η^2-(η^2-$C_5H_{10}O_2$)P{OCH (CO OMe)CH(COOMe)O}P(η^2-$C_5H_{10}O_2$)}$(Cl)_2$] [24], and [Pt{η^2-(η^2-$C_{17}H_{16}$ NO_2)P{OCH(Ph)CH(Ph)O}P(η^2-$C_{17}H_{16}NO_2$)]$(Cl)_2$].4$CHCl_3$ (at 150K) [25]. Structure of [Pt{η^2-(η^2-$C_5H_{10}O_2$)P{OCH. (COOMe)CH(COOMe)O}P(η^2-

$C_5H_{10}O_2$)}(Cl)$_2$] [24] is shown in Figure 2 as an example. Each homobidentate -P,P' donor ligand creates seven-membered metallocyclic rings of the POC_2OP type. The mean Pt-L bond distances are 2.221 Å (L = P) and 2.362 Å (Cl). The mean values of cis-L-Pt-L bond angles open in the order: 87.2° (Cl-Pt-P) < 88.2° (Cl-Pt-Cl) < 97.4° (P-Pt-P). The mean values of trans-Cl-Pt-P bond angle are 174.3°.

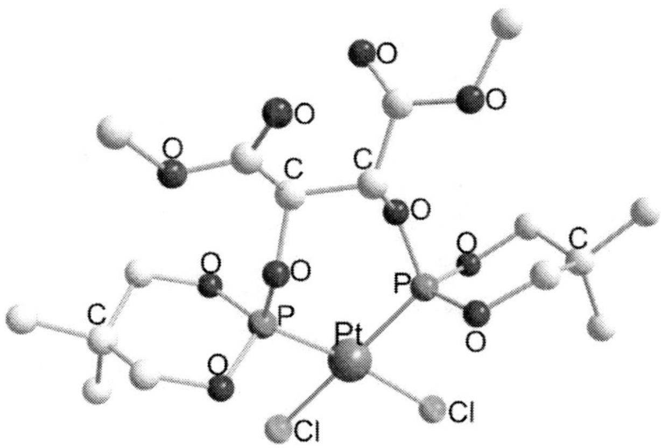

Figure 2. Structure of [Pt{η^2-(η^2-$C_5H_{10}O_2$)P{OCH(COOMe)CH(COOMe)O}P(η^2-$C_5H_{10}O_2$)}(Cl)$_2$] [24].

2.3. Pt(η^2-PNC_2NP)Cl_2 Type

There are five examples of this type, which crystallized in two crystal systems: orthorhombic (1 example) and monoclinic (4 examples). Such complexes are: [Pt{η^2-Ph_2P(2,2'-bipyrrolidine)PPh_2}(Cl)$_2$] [26], [Pt{η^2-Ph_2P{N(CH_2Ph)CH_2CH_2($PhCH_2$)N}PPh_2}(Cl)$_2$] [27], [Pt{η^2-Pr^i_2P{N(CH_2Ph)CH_2CH_2N(CH_2Ph)}PPr^i_2(Cl)$_2$] (at 123K) [28], [Pt{η^2-(η^2-$C_4H_{10}N_2$)P{N(Me)(CH_2CH_2)N(Me)}P(η^2-$C_4H_{10}N_2$)}(Cl)$_2$] [29], and [Pt{η^2-Et_2NP(η^2-($N_2C_9H_9O$)$_2$$PNEt_2$}(Cl)$_2$].2$COCl_3$ (at 173K) [30]. Structure of [Pt{η^2-Pr^i_2P{N(CH_2Ph)CH_2CH_2N(CH_2Ph)}PPr^i_2(Cl_2)] [28] is shown in Figure 3 as an example. Each organodiphosphine ligand creates PNC_2NP metallocycles with the mean bite angle value of 96.5°. The mean values of the remaining L-Pt-L bond angles are: 87.3° (Cl-Pt-Cl), 86.9° and 172.8°

(Cl-Pt-P). The mean values of Pt-L bond distance are 2.235 Å (L = P) and 2.360 Å (Cl).

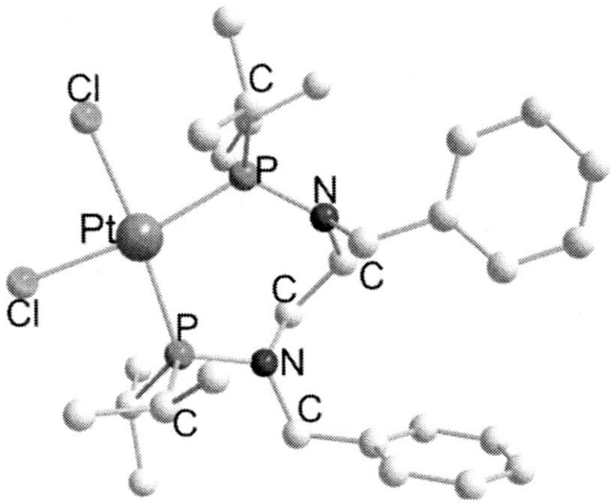

Figure 3. Structure of [Pt{η^2-Pr^i_2P{N(CH_2Ph) CH_2CH_2N(CH_2Ph)}$PPr^i_2$$(Cl)_2$] [28].

2.4. Pt(η^2-PSC_2SP)Cl_2 Type

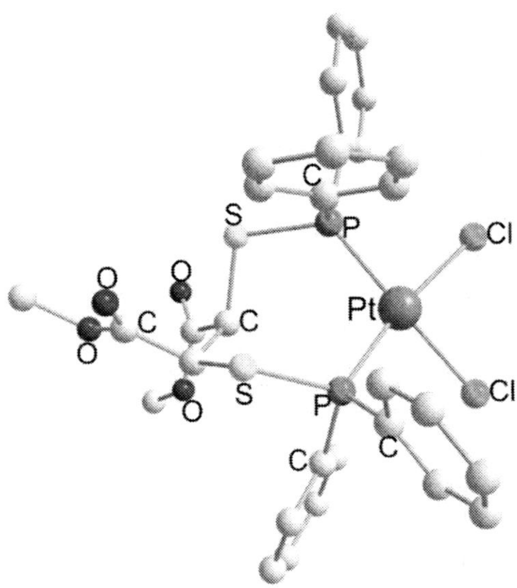

Figure 4. Structure of [Pt{η^2-Ph_2P{SC(COOMe)C(COOMe)S}PPh_2}$(Cl)_2$] [31].

Triclinic [Pt{η^2-Ph_2P{SC(COOMe)C(COOMe)S}PPh_2}$(Cl)_2$].0.5CH_2Cl_2 (Figure 4) [31] is only example of such type. The value of PSC_2SP bite angle is 96.4°. The value of Cl-Pt-Cl bond angle is 87.7° and the mean values of cis- and trans-Cl-Pt-P bond angles are 87.7 and 172.5°, respectively.

2.5. Pt(η^2-PNC_2OP)Cl_2 Type

There are five examples of such type. The orthorhombic [Pt{η^2-$Ph_2P(NC_5H_9O)PPh_2$}$(Cl)_2$] exists in two isomeric forms [32,33], monoclinic [Pt{η^2-$Ph_2P(NC_5H_9O)Pcy_2$}$(Cl)_2$] (contains two independent molecules) [34], triclinic [Pt{η^2-Ph_2P{N(Me)CH_2CH_2O}PPh_2}$(Cl)_2$] (at 193K) [35], and orthorhombic [Pt{η^2-(η^2-$C_{12}H_{18}O_2$)$P(NC_5H_9O)P$(η^2-$C_{12}H_{18}O_2$)} $(Cl)_2$]. CH_2Cl_2 [36].

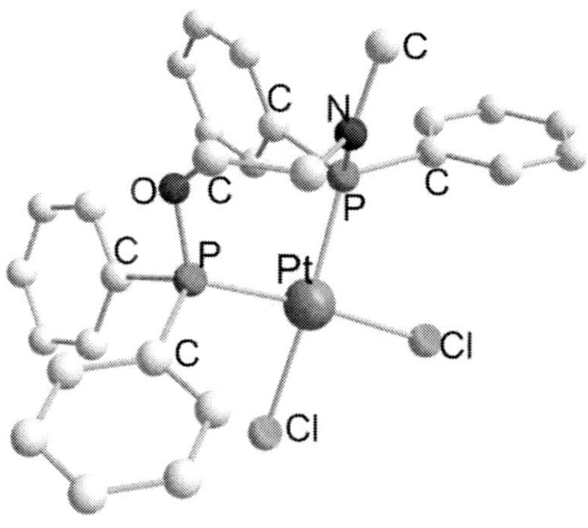

Figure 5. Structure of [Pt{η^2-Ph_2P{N(Me)CH_2CH_2O}PPh_2}$(Cl)_2$] [35].

Structure of [Pt{η^2-Ph_2P{N(Me)CH_2CH_2O}PPh_2}$(Cl)_2$] [35] is shown in Figure 5 as an example. Each organodisphosphine ligand creates seven-membered metallocyclic ring (PNC_2OP). The values of P-Pt-P bite angles in two isomers are 95.1° [32] and 95.3° [33]. The mean Pt-L bond distances are 2.234 Å (L = P) and 2.354 Å (Cl) in [32] and 2.236 Å (L = P) and 2.343 Å (Cl) in [33]. Two crystallographically independent molecules within the same crystal in [34] are differ from each other of the L-Pt-L bond angles with the values (molecule 1 vs molecule 2): 99.3° (P-Pt-P), 88.0° (Cl-Pt-Cl), 86.5° (Cl-Pt-P) vs 98.9°, 87.8 and 86.7°. The mean Pt-L bond distances (molecule 1 vs molecule 2) are: 2.224 Å (L = P) and 2.358 Å (Cl) vs 2.224 Å and 2.354 Å. The isomers as well as the independent molecules are examples of distortion isomers [37].

The comprehensive mean values of cis-L-Pt-L bond angles in [32-36] open in the sequence: 87.3° (Cl-Pt-P) < 88.2° (Cl-Pt-Cl) < 97.2° (P-Pt-P). The mean value of trans-Cl-Pt-P bond angles is 174.5°. The total mean values of Pt-L bond distances are 2.227 Å (L = P) and 2.352 Å (Cl).

CONCLUSION

This review covers over thirty examples of cis-PtP_2Cl_2 derivatives in which organodiphosphines create seven-membered metallocyclic rings. These complexes crystallized in three crystal classes: triclinic (6 examples), orthorhombic (12 examples) and monoclinic (16 examples). The organodiphosphine ligands create the following seven-membered metallocycles: PC_4P, (most common), PNC_2NP, POC_2OP, PSC_2SP and $PtNC_2OP$. The comprehensive mean values of cis- L-Pt-L bond angles open in the sequences: 87.3° (Cl-Pt-Cl) < 87.7° (Cl-Pt-P) < 96.8° (P-Pt-P). The mean trans-Cl-Pt-P bond angle is 173.5°.

The orthorhombic $[Pt\{\eta^2\text{-}Ph_2P(NC_5H_9O)PPh_2\}(Cl)_2]$ which exists in two isomeric forms [32, 33] and monoclinic $[Pt\{\eta^2\text{-}Ph_2P(NC_5H_9O)Pcy_2\}(Cl)_2]$ which contains two crystllographically independent molecules within the same crystal [34] are classical examples of distortion isomers [6].

Comprehensive mean values of selected structural parameters in cis-PtP_2Cl_2 derivatives with various metallocycles are summarized in Table 1. As can be seen there is cooperative effects between cis-L-Pt-L bond angles, the P-Pt-P bite angles growing with the size of metallocyclic ring and the remaining cis-Cl-Pt-Cl and cis-P-Pt-Cl bond angles closes. The sum of all four (Pt-P (x2) + Pt-Cl (x2)) bond distances smoothly growing with the size of the respective metallocycles.

Table 1. Comprehensive mean values of selected structural parameters in cis- PtP_2Cl_2 derivatives

Metallocyclic ring (number of examples)	P-Pt-P [°]	Cl-Pt-Cl [°]	P-Pt-Cl [°]	Pt-P [Å]	Pt-Cl [Å]	Pt-L (x4) [Å]
four-membered[a] (24 examples)	72.4	91.7	97.3 170.4	2.214	2.352	9.13
five-membered[a] (31 examples)	86.4	88.0	92.7 175.7	2.216	2.354	9.14
six-membered[b] (42 examples)	94.0	87.6	89.0 175.6	2.222	2.358	9.16
seven-membered[c] (34 examples)	96.8	87.3	87.0 173.5	2.239	2.346	9.17

Ref. [2].
Ref. [3].
This work.

ACKNOWLEDGMENTS

This work was supported by the projects VEGA 1/0873/15, KEGA 022UK-4/2015, APVV-15-0585.

REFERENCES

[1] Melník M., Mikuš P., Organomonophosphines in PtP_2Cl_2 derivatives: structural aspects. *Rev. Inorg. Chem.,* 2015, *35*, pp 179-189.

[2] Melník M., Forgácsová A. and Mikuš P., Organodiphosphines in cis-Pt(η^2-PXP)$(Cl)_2$ and cis-Pt(η^2-PXXP)$(Cl)_2$ Derivatives – Structural Aspects. *New Developments in Oncology Research*, Nova Science Publ. Inc., NY, USA, 2018, Chapter 1.

[3] Melník M., Forgácsová A. and Mikuš P., Organodiphosphines in cis-Pt(η^2-PXXXP)Cl_2 Derivatives – Structural Aspects. *New Developments in Oncology Research*, Nova Science Publ. Inc., NY, USA, 2018, Chapter 2

[4] Gramlich V., Consiglio G., Crystal Structures of the (−)-DIOP Complexes of Nickel, Palladium and Platinum Dichloride. *Helv. Chim. Acta*, 1979, *62*, pp 1016-1024.

[5] Ganter C., Orpen A. G., Bergamini P., Costa E., A new orthorhombic crystal form of dichloro[(–)-(*R*,*R*)-2,2-dimethyl-4,5-bis(diphenyl phosphinomethyl)-1,3-dioxolane-*P*,*P*']platinum, [{(*R*,*R*)-diop}$PtCl_2$]. *Acta Crystallogr., Sect. C,* 1994, *50*, pp 507-510.

[6] Melník M., Holloway C. E., Stereochemistrfy of platinum coordination compounds, *Coord. Chem. Rev.,* 2006, *250,* 2261-2270.

[7] Deacon G. B., Elliott P. W., Erven A. P., Meyer G., The Synthesis by Decarboxylation Reactions and Crystal Structures of 1, n–Bis(diphenylphosphino)alkane(pentafluorophenyl)-platinum(II) Complexes, *Z. Anorg. Allg. Chem*., 2005, *631*, pp 843-850.

[8] Watson W. H., Huang S. H., Wang L., Richmond M. G., Ligand Substitution Chemistry of the Diphosphine Ligand *endo,endo*-2,3-Bis(diphenylphosphinomethyl)-5-norbornene (dpmn): Syntheses and X-ray Diffraction Structures of $PtCl_2$(dmn) and $PtMe_2$(dpmn). *J. Chem. Cryst*., 2009, *39*, pp 740-746.

[9] Doherty S., Robins E. G, Nieuwenhuyzen M., Knight J. G., Champkin P. A., Clegg W., Synthesis of a New Class of 1,4-Bis (diphenylphosphino)-1,3-butadiene Bridged Diphosphine, NUPHOS, via Zirconium-Mediated Reductive Coupling of Alkynes and Diynes: Applications in Palladium-Catalyzed Cross-Coupling Reactions. *Organometallics,* 2002, *21,* pp 1383-1399.

[10] Fanjul T., Eastham G., Fey N., Hamilton A., Orpen A. G., Pringle P. G., Waugh M., Palladium Complexes of the Heterodiphosphine *o*-$C_6H_4(CH_2P^tBu_2)(CH_2PPh_2)$ Are Highly Selective and Robust Catalysts for the Hydromethoxycarbonylation of Ethene. *Organometallics,* 2010, *29*, pp 2292-2305.

[11] Fanjul T., Eastham G., Floure J., Forrest S. J. K., Haddow M. F., Hamilton A., Pringle P. G., Orpen A. G., Waugh M., Interplay of bite angle and cone angle effects. A comparison between *o*-C_6H_4 $(CH_2PR_2)(PR'_2)$ and*o*-$C_6H_4(CH_2PR_2)(CH_2PR'_2)$ as ligands for Pd-

catalysed ethene hydromethoxycarbonylation. *Dalton Trans.*, 2013, *42*, pp 100-115.

[12] Doherty S., Knight J. J., Smyth C. H., Hanington R. W., Clegg W., Biaryl-Like CATPHOS Diphosphines via Double Diels–Alder Cycloaddition between 1,4-Bis(diphenylphosphinoyl)buta-1,3-diyne and Anthracenes: Efficient Ligands for the Palladium-Catalyzed Amination of Aromatic Bromides and α-Arylation of Ketones. *Organometallics,* 2008, *27*, pp 1679-1682.

[13] Doherty S., Goodrich P., Hardacre C., Luo H. K., Nieuwenhuyzen M., Rath R. K., Lewis Acid Platinum Complexes of Conformationally Flexible NUPHOS Diphosphines: Highly Efficient Catalysts for the Carbonyl−Ene Reaction. *Organometallics*, 2005, *24*, pp 5945-5955.

[14] Doherty S., Knight J. G., Smyth C. H., Harrington R. W., Clegg W., Asymmetric Platinum Group Metal-Catalyzed Carbonyl-Ene Reactions: Carbon−Carbon Bond Formation versus Isomerization. *J. Org. Chem.*, 2006, *71*, pp 9751-9764.

[15] Mikami K., Kakuno H., Aikawe K., Enantiodiscrimination and Enantiocontrol of Neutral and Cationic Pt^{II} Complexes Bearing the *Tropos* Biphep Ligand: Application to Asymmetric Lewis Acid Catalysis. *Angew. Chem. Int. Ed.,* 2005, *44*, pp 7257-7260.

[16] Weng J. F., Hong W., Yan K., Mak T. C. W., Wong H. N. C., Synthesis, Resolution, and Applications of 1,16-Dihydroxy-tetraphenylene as a Novel Building Block in Molecular Recognition and Assembly. *J. Org. Chem.*, 2003, *68*, pp 8918-8931.

[17] Doherty S., Knight J. G., Smyth C. H., Harrington R. W., Clegg W., Rhodium-Catalyzed Double [2 + 2 + 2] Cycloaddition of 1,4-Bis(diphenylphosphinoyl)buta-1,3-diyne with Tethered Diynes: A Modular, Highly Versatile Single-Pot Synthesis of NU-BIPHEP Biaryl Diphosphines. *Org. Lett.*, 2007, *9*, pp 4925-4928.

[18] Petzold H., Alzawashdeh A. I. S., Heider S., Haufe L., Ruffer T., Synthesis of 6,6′-Bis(dimethylamino)- and 6,6′-Dibromo-Substituted 2,2′-Diphosphanylbiphenyls and Their Palladium Complexes. *Eur. J. Inorg. Chem.*, 2013, pp 4858-4866.

[19] Benicezi T., Rizro S., Pilati T., Ponti A., Sado M., Pagliarisie E., Rarri S., Giuseppe C., de Ferra L., Sannicolo F., Process-scale preparation of enantiomerically pure γ-lactones by asymmetric hydrogenation of γ-ketoesters and comparative tests of the sensory properties of some antipodes. *Tetrahedron Asymm.*, 2004, *15*, pp 2289-2297.

[20] Edwards P. G., Knight J. C., Newman P. D., Synthesis of (1*R*,4*S*,6*R*)-5,5,6-trimethyl-2-phosphabicyclo[2.2.2]octane and derivatives. *Dalton Trans.*, 2010, *39*, pp 3851-3860.

[21] Bergamini P., Bertolasi V., Cattabridgea M., Ferretti V., Loprieno U., Mantovani N., Marvello L., Template Synthesis of Chiral Vicinal Diphosphinites as Their Pt^{II} and Pd^{II} Complexes. *Eur. J. Inorg. Chem.*, 2003, pp 918-925.

[22] Sharma R. K., Samuelson A. G., Asymmetric allylation of aldehydes with chiral platinum phosphinite complexes. *Tetrahedron Asymm.*, 2007, *18*, pp 2387-2393.

[23] Bergamini P., Bertolasi V., Milani F., The Construction of P-O/P-N Ligands on Platinum and Palladium, *Eur. J. Inorg. Chem.*, 2004, pp 1277-1284.

[24] Orvens Jr. S. B., Gray G. M., Synthesis, characterization, and coordination chemistry of two new tartaric acid-derived bis(phosphite) ligands. *J. Organomet. Chem.*, 2008, *693*, pp 3907-3914.

[25] Clochard M., Mattmann E., Mercier F., Ricard L., Mathey F., Phosphinites Derived from the 7-Phosphanorbornene Skeleton: First Results in Asymmetric Catalysis. *Org. Lett.,* 2003, *5*, pp 3093-3094.

[26] Meäzenberg R., Rademacher P., Boese R., Chiral platinum (II) complexes with phosphorus derivatives of the amino acid l-proline. NMR spectroscopic and X-ray structure investigations of the cis influence of tertiary phosphorus ligands. *J. Mol. Struct.*, 1998, *444*, pp 77-90.

[27] Balakrishna M. S., Abhyankar R. M., Mague J. T., New bis(phosphines) derived from *N,N* '-substituted ethylenediamine derivatives. Synthesis and transition metal chemistry of $X_2PN(R)$ $CH_2CH_2(R)NPX_2$ (R = CH_2Ph or Ph, X = Ph; R = CH_2Ph, X_2 = $O_2C_6H_4$). The crystal and molecular structure of $Ph_2PN(CH_2Ph)$

$CH_2CH_2(CH_2Ph)NPPh_2$ and cis-[{$PtCl_2Ph_2PN(CH_2Ph)CH_2CH_2$ (CH_2 Ph) $NPPh_2$}] *J. Chem. Soc., Dalton Trans.*, 1999, pp 1407-1412.

[28] Zubiri M. R., Nielton H. L., Cole-Hamilton D. J., Slawin A. M. Z., Woollins J. D., Bis(phosphine) derivatives of diamines. *Polyhedron,* 2004, *23*, pp 693-699.

[29] Powell J., Lough A., Raso M., Synthesis, structure and relative hydrolytic stability of *cis*-[$PtCl_2L$] and *cis*-[$W(CO)_4L$] where L is the bidentate triaminophosphine ligand [$MeNCH_2CH_2N(Me)PN(Me)CH_2$]$_2$. *J. Chem. Soc., Dalton Trans.*, 1994, pp 1571-1576.

[30] Tei Z., Thonnesen H., Jones P. G., Crowe L., Harris R. K., Schmutzler R., Alkyl-Tethered Bis-Phosphoryl Compounds with two 1,3,2-Benzodiazaphosphorinone Units; Oxidation, Complexation, and X-Ray Structure Analysis of Selected Compounds. *Z. Anorg. Allg. Chem.,* 2000, *626*, pp 1763-1772.

[31] Bergamini P., Bertolasi V., Giordani R., Platinum-assisted preparation of PS ligands containing chiral centress; X-ray crystal structure of a dithiophosphinite platínum complex, *Inorg. Chim. Acta*, 2005, *358*, pp 2031-2039.

[32] Bandini A. L., Banditelli G., Cesarotti E., Mainghetti G., Bovio B., Mono- and dinuclear complexes of platinum(II) with chiral diphosphines: Pt(P-P')Cl2 and [Pt(P-P')(.mu.-OH)]2[BF4]2(P-P'=prolophos, N-(diphenylphosphino)-2-((diphenylphoshpinoxy) methyl) pyrrolidine, and butaphos, 1-(diphenylphosphinoxy)-2-(N-ethyl-N-(diphenylphosphino)amino)butane). Crystal and molecular structure of P{S-prolophos-P,P'}Cl2. *Inorg. Chem.*, 1992, *31*, pp 391-398.

[33] Naili S., Carpentier J. F., Agbossou G., Mortreux A., Nowogrocki G., Wignacourt J. P., Platinum(II) Aminophosphine- and Amido-phosphine-Phosphinite Complexes: Synthesis, Structure, and Use in Catalytic Asymmetric Hydroformylation of Styrene. Crystal Structure of [(S)-1-(Diphenylphosphino)-2-(((diphenylphosphino)oxy) methyl) pyrrolidine]dichloro platinum(II). *Organometllics*, 1995, *14*, pp 401-406.

[34] Naili S., Carpentier J. F., Agbossou F., Mortreux A., Nowogrocki G., Wignacourt J. P., Ligand effect on the insertion of $SnCl_2$ in dichloroplatinum(II) complexes of symmetrical and mixed amino(do)phosphine phosphinite chelates - X-Ray crystal structure of $PtCl_2$((S)-Ph,Cy-PRONOP). *New J. Chem.*, 1997, *21*, pp 919-927.

[35] Balakrishna M. S., Mc Donald P., Synthesis, spectroscopic study and X-ray crystal structure of unsymmetrical bis(phosphine)-platinum complex, [PtCl2{η2-Ph2POCH2CH2N(CH3)PPh2]. *Inorg. Chem. Commun.*, 2002, *5*, pp 782-786.

[36] Naili S., Suisse I., Mortreux A., Agbossou-Niederoom F., Nowogrocki G., Chiral aminophosphonite-phosphite ligands: synthesis and use in platinum- and rhodium-based enantioselective hydroformylation of styrene. Crystal structure of [(S)-N-(2,2′biphenoxyphosphino)-2-(2,2′biphenoxyphosphinoxymethyl)pyrrolidine]dichloro platinum(II). *J. Organomet. Chem.*, 2001, *628*, pp 114-122.

INDEX

B

C

D

E

D

E

I

J

K

L

M

N

O

P

Q

R

S

T

U

V

W

Z

Oncology: The Promising Future of Biomarkers

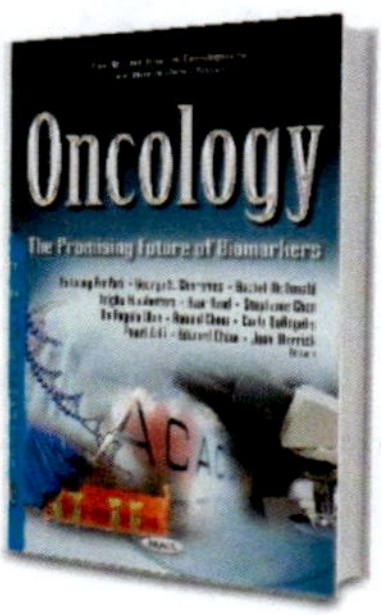

Editors: Anthony Furfari, M.D., George S. Charames, Rachel McDonald, Leigha Rowbottom, Azar Azad, Stephanie Chan, Bo Angela Wan, Ronald Chow, Carlo DeAngelis, Pearl Zaki, Edward Chow, Ph.D., and Joav Merrick, M.D., MMedSci, DMSc

Series: Health and Human Development

Book Description: In this book, the authors synthesize existing biomarker research in the literature related to cancer and the potential effect it may have on future treatment, drug metabolism, symptom burden, radiation response, susceptibility to radiation related toxicities, and prognosis.

Hardcover ISBN: 978-1-53610-608-4
Retail Price: $195

Horizons in Cancer Research. Volume 71

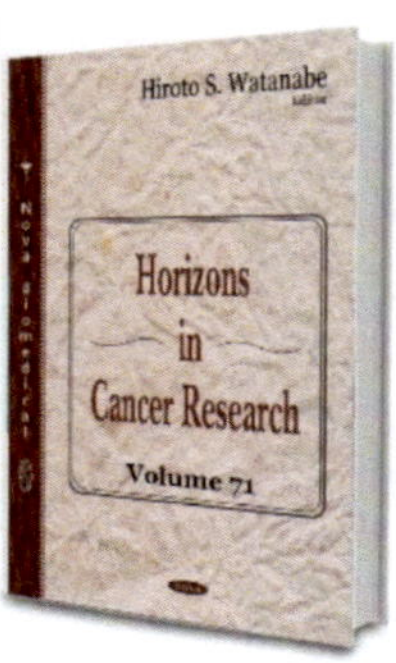

Editor: Hiroto S. Watanabe

Series: Horizons in Cancer Research

Book Description: Horizons in Cancer Research. Volume 71 begins by reviewing the histopathological features of head and neck squamous cell carcinoma and its precursor lesions, risk factors for head and neck squamous cell carcinoma including viral infection, chemical carcinogenic and ethnic predisposition.

Hardcover ISBN: 978-1-53615-207-4
Retail Price: $250